Practical Medical Procedures

at a Glance

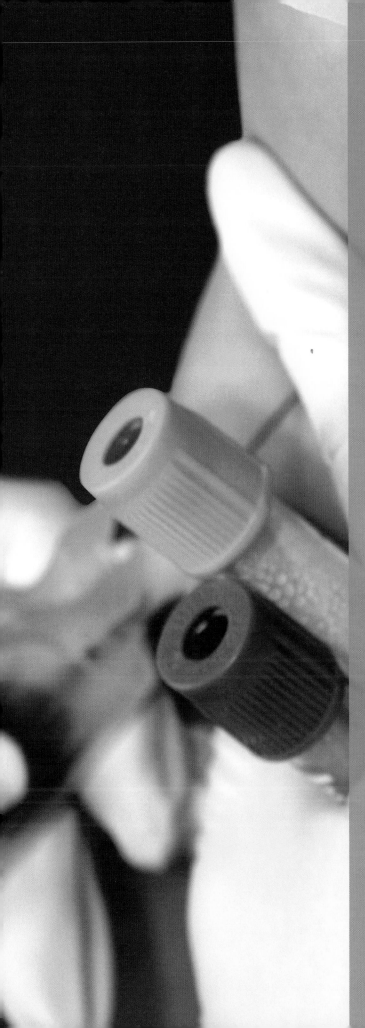

Practical Medical Procedures

at a Glance

Rachel K. Thomas, BM, BCh, BEng (Hons), BSc
South Thames Foundation programme
London, UK

With contributions from:

Catherine J. Taylor, BM, BCh, PhD, BSc (Hons)
South East Scotland Foundation programme
Edinburgh, UK

Aletta E. Richards, MB, BCh, DA, FCA
Consultant Anaesthetist
Oxford Universities NHS Trust
Clinical Skills Tutor
Division of Medical Sciences,
The University of Oxford, UK

Diana E. Thomas, BSc (Hons), PhD
Scientific Director
Centre for Evidence Based Paediatrics,
Gastroenterology and Nutrition
Sydney Medical School, The University
KRI, The Children's Hospital at Westmead
Sydney, NSW, Australia

WILEY Blackwell

A John Wiley & Sons, Ltd., Publication

Registered Office   John Wiley & Sons Ltd, The Atrium, Southern Gate, Chichester, West Sussex, PO19 8SQ, UK

Editorial Offices   350 Main Street, Malden, MA 02148-5020, USA
9600 Garsington Road, Oxford, OX4 2DQ, UK
The Atrium, Southern Gate, Chichester, West Sussex, PO19 8SQ, UK

For details of our global editorial offices, for customer services, and for information about how to apply for permission to reuse the copyright material in this book please see our website at www.wiley.com/wiley-blackwell.

Library of Congress Cataloging-in-Publication Data
Thomas, Rachel Katherine, author.
  Practical medical procedures at a glance / Rachel Katherine Thomas, Catherine Jane Taylor, Aletta Elizabeth Richards, Diana Elizabeth Thomas.
       p. ; cm.
  Includes bibliographical references and index.
    ISBN 978-1-118-63285-7 (paper)
  I. Taylor, Catherine Jane, author.   II. Richards, Aletta Elizabeth, author.   III. Thomas, Diana Elizabeth, author.   IV. Title.
    [DNLM: 1. Clinical Medicine–methods–Practice Guideline.   2. Clinical Competence–standards–Practice Guideline. WB 102]
  RC55
  616–dc23
                                                                2014048462

A catalogue record for this book is available from the British Library.

Cover image: Reproduced from iStock © Bryngelzon

Set in Minion Pro 9.5/11.5 by Aptara
Printed and bound in Singapore by Markono Print Media Pte Ltd

1 2015

Contents

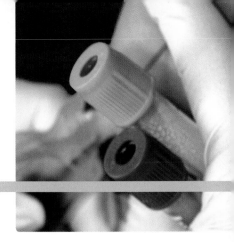

Preface   vii
Acknowledgements   viii
About the companion website   ix
How to use your textbook   x

Part 1 **Introduction**   **1**
1   Overview of practical procedures   2
2   Non-technical skills   4
3   Waste, sharps disposal and injuries   6

Part 2 **Common preliminary components**   **9**
4   Identifying a patient   10
5   Consent, capacity and documentation   12
6   Hand hygiene and personal protective equipment   14
7   Scrubbing in   16
8   Asepsis   18

Part 3 **Common non-invasive ward procedures**   **21**
9   Measuring vital signs   22
10   Writing a safe prescription   24

Part 4 **Common invasive ward procedures**   **27**
11   Performing venepuncture   28
12   Taking blood cultures   30
13   Inserting a cannula in a peripheral vein   32
14   Measuring blood glucose   34
15   Suturing   36

Part 5 **Administering medications**   **39**
16   Administering intravenous infusions   40
17   Administering intravenous infusions of blood and
     blood products   42
18   Administering parenteral medications   44
19   Administering injections   46

Part 6 **Common procedures – respiratory**   **49**
20   Measuring arterial blood gas   50
21   Administering oxygen therapy   52
22   Using inhalers and nebulisers   54

23 Assessing respiratory function 56
24 Using airway manoeuvres and simple adjuncts 58
25 Ventilating with a bag valve mask device 60

Part 7

Common procedures – cardiology 63

26 Recording a 12-lead electrocardiogram 64
27 Performing cardiopulmonary resuscitation 66

Part 8

Common procedures – gastroenterology 69

28 Inserting a nasogastric tube 70
29 Performing a digital rectal examination 72

Part 9

Common procedures – urology 75

30 Performing urinalysis 76
31 Inserting a bladder catheter 78

Part 10

Common procedures – otolaryngology 81

32 Performing otoscopy 82

Part 11

Common procedures – ophthalmology 85

33 Performing ophthalmoscopy 86

Part 12

Common procedures – end-of-life care 89

34 Confirming and certifying death 90

Part 13

Supplementary resources 93

Multiple choice questions 94
Answers to multiple choice questions 104
Further reading and references 114
Index 117

Preface

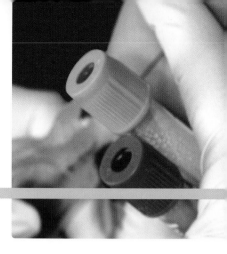

Practical procedures are an integral part of many clinical encounters. They are a mainstay of good clinical care. Accordingly, regulatory bodies such as the General Medical Council now require procedures to be formally recognised and assessed as a prerequisite to gaining full registration.

The intention of this book is to provide a resource to help guide in the safe and effective acquisition of these skills. It is intended to supplement the teaching provided by a multitude of experienced clinicians – the doctors, nurses, site practitioners, professors, medical school tutors and lecturers – not to replace it. Each skill or procedure possesses protocols specific to each Healthcare Trust or region of practice which, of course, must be adhered to first and foremost.

The online representations of the procedures are included to help readers understand the practical aspects of the procedures – but, as with any skill, there is no replacement for repetition.

The suggested further reading and references are included as they have been consulted in the writing of this book, and they are valuable resources to further expand upon its contents.

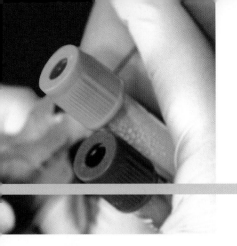

Acknowledgements

Many minds have contributed to the formation of this book. Appreciation is shown to the contributors, Dr Aletta Elizabeth Richards and Dr Catherine Jane Taylor, for their contributions to the book: Dr Richards for her overall support of the book and for assistance with content, images and videography; and Dr Taylor for her contributions to Chapters 8, 14, 21–25, 27 and 29–33.

I appreciate the invaluable assistance of Dr Diana Elizabeth Thomas for extensive reviewing and editing of the manuscript, and to Hugh Thomas for his support. Special thanks go to Camilla Thomas, for her continuous and tireless assistance and enthusiasm throughout the entire project. Without her, this book would not exist.

Thanks to Jon Story for assistance with images and Eoghan Synnot with editing and videography. Thanks to Quentin Deluge for help with sound. Thanks are also extended to James, Andrew, and Matthew Thomas, Jack Russell, Rosalie Brooman-White, Joshua Luck and Alix Brazier for assistance with images.

Thanks to Khadar Abdul for his assistance at the clinical skills laboratory at the University of Oxford.

Thanks to Elizabeth Johnson, Katrina Rimmer, Fiona Goodgame, Andrew Hallam and their colleagues at Wiley Blackwell, as well as Amit Malik at Aptara, for their expertise, advice and support.

Thanks are also extended to the medical students and junior and senior doctors who made time to review manuscripts in the early stages of the book – your feedback has been greatly appreciated.

About the companion website

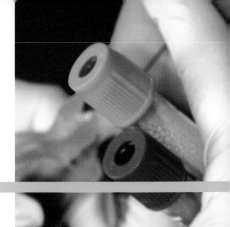

Don't forget to visit the companion website for this book:

www.ataglanceseries.com/ practicalmedprocedures

There you will find valuable material designed to enhance your learning, including:

- Interactive multiple choice questions
- Videos demonstrating practical techniques

Scan this QR code to visit the companion website:

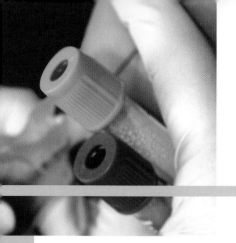

How to use your textbook

Features contained within your textbook

Each topic is presented in a double-page spread with clear, easy-to-follow diagrams supported by succinct explanatory text.

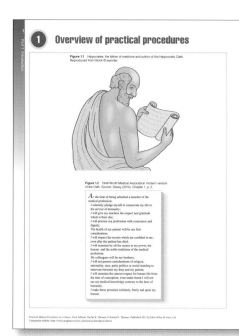

Hints and tips boxes give inside information on a topic.

Hints and tips:
- **First, do no harm!**
- Don't hesitate to ask for **help**.
- **Document** your actions – successful or otherwise.
- Take care to **not injure yourself** when **moving patients** – used approved **aids** and **methods**.
- Follow **local protocols**.
- **Keep up** with **best current practice**.

Did you know boxes highlight points to remember.

Your textbook is full of **photographs, illustrations and tables.**

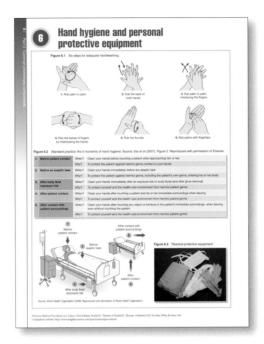

Multiple choice **questions,** at the end of the book and followed by the answers, help you test yourself.

The website icon indicates that you can read more on a topic by visiting the companion website. / **The website icon** indicates that you can find accompanying resources on the book's companion website.

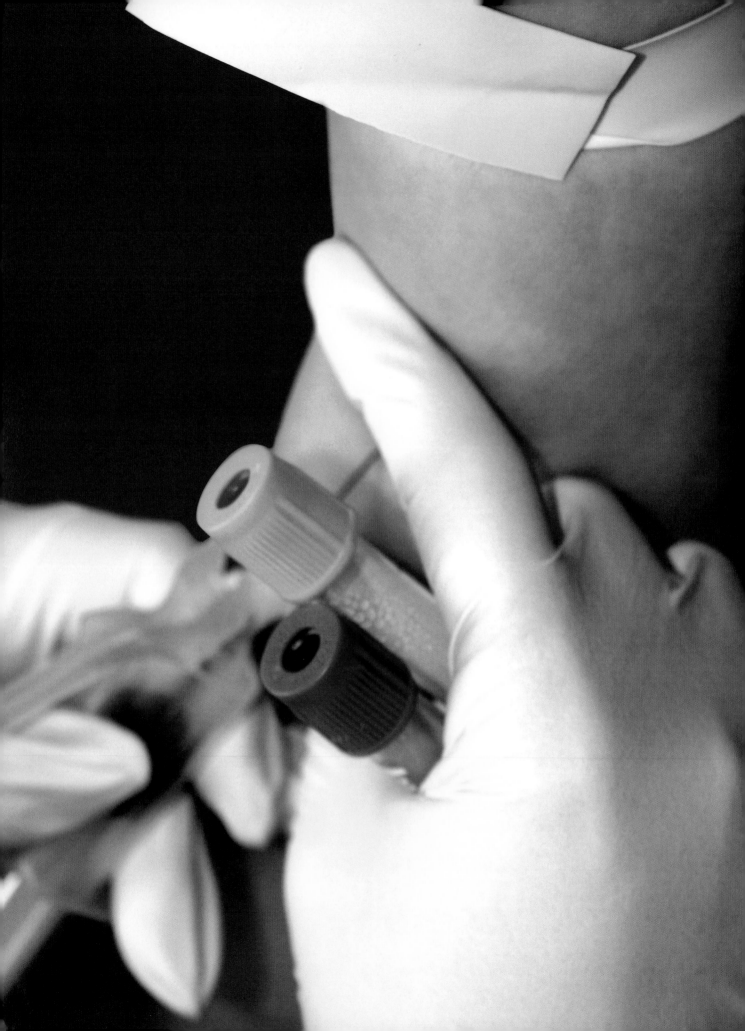

Introduction

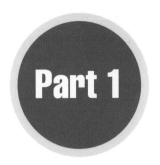

Part 1

Chapters

1   Overview of practical procedures   2
2   Non-technical skills   4
3   Waste, sharps disposal and injuries   6

① Overview of practical procedures

Figure 1.1 Hippocrates: the father of medicine and author of the Hippocratic Oath. Reproduced from iStock © wynnter.

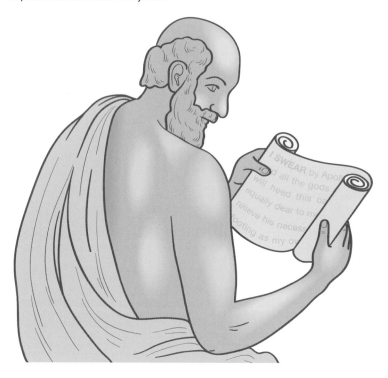

Figure 1.2 1948 World Medical Association modern version of the Oath. Source: Davey (2014), Chapter 1, p. 2.

*A*t the time of being admitted a member of the medical profession:

I solemnly pledge myself to consecrate my life to the service of humanity;

I will give my teachers the respect and gratitude which is their due;

I will practise my profession with conscience and dignity;

*T*he health of my patient will be my first consideration;

I will respect the secrets which are confided in me, even after the patient has died;

I will maintain by all the means in my power, the honour and the noble traditions of the medical profession;

*M*y colleagues will be my brothers;

I will not permit considerations of religion, nationality, race, party politics or social standing to intervene between my duty and my patient;

I will maintain the utmost respect for human life from the time of conception; even under threat I will not use my medical knowledge contrary to the laws of humanity.

I make these promises solemnly, freely and upon my honour.

Practical Medical Procedures at a Glance, First Edition. Rachel K. Thomas © Rachel K. Thomas. Published 2015 by John Wiley & Sons, Ltd.
Companion website: http://www.ataglanceseries.com/practicalmedprocedures

What are practical procedures?

The **practical procedures** addressed in this book, and in the **online learning materials**, are a group of processes that medical practitioners are required to be **proficient** in.

Whilst these requirements may shift, varying with different regulatory bodies, Healthcare Trusts and local protocols, most of the included procedures are part of the current recommendation of required skills by the **General Medical Council (GMC).**

Why are they important?

Proficiency is required in order to contribute to **quality patient care** – facilitating the provision of a more beneficial clinical encounter for both the patient and the medical practitioner. Many of these skills are staple components of daily life in most hospitals, as they are required for the **diagnosis** and **management** of a vast range of medical conditions.

Furthermore, proficiency in these skills is part of the **current requirements** for doctors to gain their full medical registration.

Using this resource

This book is best used when coupled with the **supplementary online learning materials**. Each chapter addresses a procedure or closely linked set of skills – **what** it is, **why** it is used, and several relevant **indications**, **contra-indications** and **complications**. As the focus of this resource is on assisting in the acquisition of skills, the information relating to indications, contra-indications and complications is by no means exhaustive. The contra-indications listed may be relative or absolute. Various other sources of information, some of which are included in the **Further reading and references** section at the back of the book, focus more fully on the pathology and medical settings of these procedures. In some skills, common **pathology** is also briefly mentioned to give some context to the procedure and its frequent findings. Most chapters include a **step-by-step** breakdown of how to perform the practical procedure. Most also include a **Hints and Tips** box with suggestions and important points to remember.

The chapters correspond to **self-assessment questions**, which are included both in the book and online. The majority of chapters also correspond to an **online video**, which shows in real time how to perform the practical procedure, and the equipment required to do so.

Proficiency in performing these procedures, as with any new skill, takes **time** and **practice**. **Repetition** is the key! Generally, it is preferable to **read** about the procedure and **how** to do it, and to then **watch** it several times, prior to attempting it yourself in a skills laboratory, if possible, before attempting it on a patient. Many skills laboratories have either low-fidelity or high-fidelity simulations to facilitate learning.

General advice

Be sure to ask for **help** from your seniors and colleagues – they also had to learn once, and thus they will usually be happy to help.

Ensure that you are not interrupting his or her clinical commitments or affecting patient care, and if you are, it may be more suitable to ask someone else.

Never attempt a procedure on a patient if you do not feel confident or capable of performing it safely – it is not appropriate to feel coerced into clinical procedures you do not feel qualified to carry out. Ensure that you have enough self-awareness and confidence to be aware of not only your **capabilities** but also your **limitations**. Remember the **Hippocratic Oath** – first, do no harm (Figures 1.1 and 1.2)! Ensure that you also look after **yourself**. Take breaks, and ensure that you eat and drink regularly, particularly during long shifts. Also ensure that you **avoid injuring yourself** by adhering to 'moving and handling' protocols, such as using **slides**, **hoists** and **approved methods** for moving patients.

As will be covered in each of the following chapters of this book, ensure that you fully and correctly **identify** the patient, and **document** your actions in the relevant areas. Usually, this will mean in the **patient notes**, although for some procedures (e.g. cannulation), some hospitals will require this to also be included on the **medication chart**. Ensure that you also document procedures that you attempted that were **not successful** – do not feel embarrassed to do so.

In many situations, **site practitioners** or **nurses** may be able to perform the procedure. Whilst at times when you are very busy, this will be a blessing, ensure that you obtain **adequate experience** in performing them too. There is no substitute for **practice** – with it the procedures will become much easier, as your **confidence** grows.

Remember that many clinical settings have clear **guidance** and **protocols** available to assist in practical procedures. Ensure that you become familiar with these as soon as possible, as they will help both you and your patients. This book's information on each practical procedure is included as guidance only – it is important to remember that **best current practice** constantly evolves, and it is the medical practitioner's responsibility to keep up with any changes as they appear. Guidance is available online from resources such as the **GMC's** *Tomorrow's Doctors*.

Finally, everyone has periods of time when they lose confidence, and are unsuccessful in procedures that had previously been mastered. This will pass – perhaps after requesting guidance from a senior to improve technique, perhaps after confidence increases or perhaps simply after luck has improved! Everyone had to learn once – you are not the first person to have trouble removing that last little air bubble from that syringe. …

Hints and tips:
- **First, do no harm!**
- Don't hesitate to ask for **help**.
- **Document** your actions – successful or otherwise.
- Take care to **not injure yourself** when **moving patients** – used approved **aids** and **methods**.
- Follow **local protocols**.
- **Keep up** with **best current practice**.

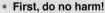

2 Non-technical skills

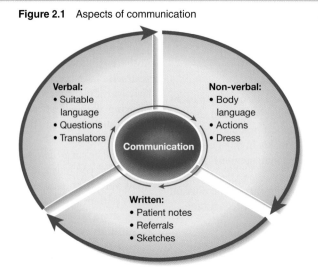

Figure 2.1 Aspects of communication

Verbal:
• Suitable language
• Questions
• Translators

Non-verbal:
• Body language
• Actions
• Dress

Communication

Written:
• Patient notes
• Referrals
• Sketches

Figure 2.2 Aspects of non-technical skills. Adapted from Fletcher G, et al, (2003).

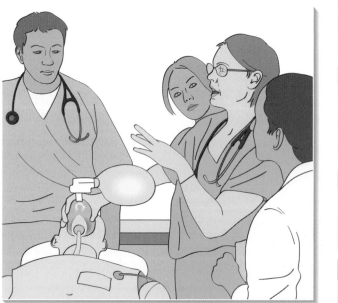

Situation awareness
• Anticipation
• Information interpretation
• Questioning
• Workspace modification

Task management
• Planning
• Preparing
• Prioritising
• Resource identification and allocation

Team working
• Leadership
• Role allocation
• Co-operation
• Communication

Decision making
• Evaluation of risks
• Evaluation of benefits
• Re-evaluation
• Modification

What are non-technical skills?

Non-technical skills are a range of skills which impact on a clinical situation, but are related to areas other than practical proficiency. They can be difficult to evaluate, relating to social, mental and personal resources. Underpinning them, to various degrees, are **communication skills**. These include **verbal** and **non-verbal** communication (Figure 2.1). Non-technical skills typically include **teamwork**, **leadership**, **situation awareness**, **task management** (including the **management of stress**) and **decision making** (Figure 2.2).

Why are they important?

These skills are important for the delivery of **good clinical care** – but, like all skills, they take time to develop. If there is a **lack** in these skills, such as poor communication within a team, uninformed decision making or illogical task management, there is an increased risk of **error**. Anticipation, effective teamwork and clear communication are examples of **good non-technical skills** which increase the chance of **optimum outcomes**.

Aspects of verbal communication

Generally, using **open-ended questions** and letting the patient talk will facilitate an interaction, after **introducing** yourself and **identifying** the patient (see Chapter 4). Request a **translator** if required. It is preferable to use a translator from an independent service (available through most Healthcare Trusts) rather than to use a patient's relative or friend – with even the most impartial intent, they may unintentionally alter aspects of the conversation, or the patient may feel pressured to alter their answers.

Use **clear sentences**, be **respectful** and have **good manners**. It is also important to establish at the outset if the patient would like a **chaperone** present, facilitating the patient's comfort (and your safety) for the rest of the clinical encounter. Ensure that you **document** having **offered** a chaperone in the patient's notes, and, if the offer was accepted, **who** was present in this role.

Always ensure that **suitable language** is used, and invite the patient to ask **questions** if they require any **clarification**. Try to establish the patient's level of **understanding** at the beginning of the interaction, to help guide you regarding what additional information is required.

Ensure that you respect patient **confidentiality**. Try to only discuss information in **appropriate areas** (such as in the doctor's office rather than in the corridor). Consider referring to patients by initials if possible, particularly if discussions risk being overheard, provided there is no confusion as to which patient is being discussed.

Ensure that conversations with patients occur in suitably **private** areas. Whilst ward curtains give the illusion of privacy, they are not soundproof! Moderate your conversation appropriately.

Aspects of non-verbal communication

Body language, the way you position your body, conveys a significant amount of information. Ensure that you have **good eye contact** with your patient, and that there are no obstacles such as computers or medical equipment in the way of this. Assume a relaxed yet **attentive posture** – avoiding positions like 'crossed arms' and 'hands on hips', as these positions can seem subtly unapproachable or excessively casual to some patients.

Actions such as **handwashing** (see Chapter 6) should be performed frequently. Perform this in the patient's view, as it reassures them that this has occurred and sets an appropriate tone for the encounter. Train yourself to do this early on, so that it becomes second nature!

Ensure that you **dress appropriately**. Neat clothing, in accordance with hospital clinical protocols (e.g. 'bare below the elbows'; see Chapter 6), is required. It is respectful of the patient, your profession and yourself to ensure that you are appropriately attired. Avoid dirty, excessively short or overly casual items of clothing.

Aspects of written communication

Written words, such as **pamphlets**, and **sketches** can also be used to help in communicating with patients. These are particularly useful at times when complex or extensive information needs to be conveyed, as the patient can review these written words as required. Also, diagrams may be useful, particularly when explaining procedures.

Patient notes are an important type of communication (see Chapter 5). It goes without saying that these documents, and any patient information, must be kept **confidential**. **Referrals** are a form of written communication that are used for formally requesting input from other practitioners. Whilst they may often be initially verbal, most referrals will require a written request. Aim to keep them **concise**, yet containing all the relevant information. Include pertinent investigations or management taken thus far – remembering that at times, important negative findings are as useful as positive findings.

Websites, including **patient support groups**, are also useful resources to help in communicating with patients.

Aspects of non-technical skills

Task management involves **prioritising** activities in order of importance, as well as **planning** and **preparing** for them in an appropriate fashion. In order to do so, **resources** need to be identified and allocated suitably. Fatigue and stress need to be recognised at times, and minimised as much as possible.

Situation awareness requires an ability to **anticipate** what may occur, after **observing**, **interpreting** and **comprehending information**. It involves actively **asking questions** to maximise understanding, and **modifying workspaces** appropriately to enable the most information to be obtained in the most effective manner.

Team working requires many aspects, such as **role allocation**, and an appreciation of the **limitations** and **capabilities** of others. It needs **co-operation**, and an ability to **communicate** information between team members effectively. It also entails **leadership** and a respect of hierarchy.

Decision making requires an appreciation of the **risks** and **benefits** of different courses of action, and the ability to **re-evaluate** selected courses and modify them appropriately.

These skills will improve over time, as both clinical exposure and medical knowledge increase. However, they are greatly facilitated by effective **communication skills**.

Hints and tips:
- Always use **appropriate language**.
- **Sketches**, **diagrams** and **written information** may help convey complex information.
- Eliciting a patient's **ideas**, **concerns** and **expectations** will enable you to provide a better clinical encounter.
- Use **open-ended questions** when speaking with patients.

3 Waste, sharps disposal and injuries

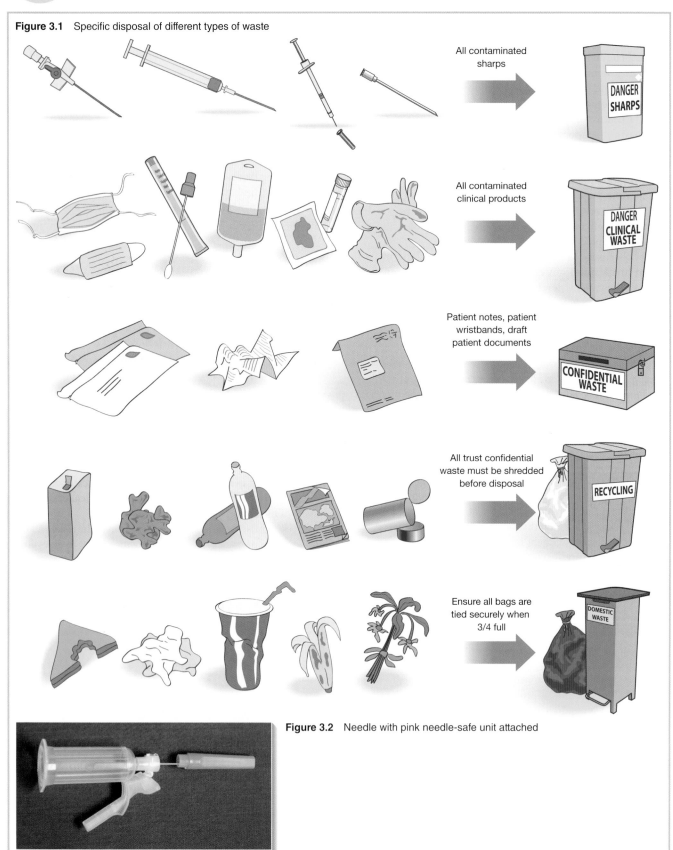

Figure 3.1 Specific disposal of different types of waste

All contaminated sharps

DANGER SHARPS

All contaminated clinical products

DANGER CLINICAL WASTE

Patient notes, patient wristbands, draft patient documents

CONFIDENTIAL WASTE

All trust confidential waste must be shredded before disposal

RECYCLING

Ensure all bags are tied securely when 3/4 full

DOMESTIC WASTE

Figure 3.2 Needle with pink needle-safe unit attached

Practical Medical Procedures at a Glance, First Edition. Rachel K. Thomas © Rachel K. Thomas. Published 2015 by John Wiley & Sons, Ltd.
Companion website: http://www.ataglanceseries.com/practicalmedprocedures

What is waste and sharps disposal?

Waste is generated in many **clinical scenarios**, and this needs to be **eliminated**. Many hospitals and trusts have strict local **protocols** on how this waste is to be disposed of. Therefore, while it may seem obvious, it is something that does require some thought. Different waste requires different disposal. **Clinical waste** must be disposed of in **clinical waste bins**, which are usually **yellow**. **Sharps** are a specific type of **clinical waste** which obviously require special care during disposal. Sharps are anything that can potentially **break the skin** – such as needles, medication ampoules, cannulae and lancets. They must be disposed of in specific **yellow clinical sharps bins**. **Domestic waste** must be disposed of in the designated bins that are usually **black**. Most clinical settings also have facilities for **recycling**. Most settings will also have a facility for **confidential waste** disposal (Figure 3.1).

Why is waste and sharps disposal important?

Obviously, waste needs to be disposed of in order to maintain **adequate cleanliness**. The need for waste to be split up into such specific groupings is due to the levels of **contamination** and **danger** associated with the disposal of the contents.

Particular care needs to be paid to the disposal of **sharps**, due to the inherent risks that they possess in causing **injury** and transmitting **bloodborne infections**. Sharps should be disposed of **immediately**. This usually involves taking a **portable sharps bin** to the site where the sharp is being used.

Clinical waste costs more to dispose of than domestic waste, as it may have **contaminated contents** such as body fluids, dressings and gloves in it. Therefore, it is important to dispose only of clinical waste in clinical waste bins.

Recycling is advisable where possible – however, great care needs to be taken to ensure that **patient confidentiality** is not breached when disposing of papers. Be sure to never throw patient lists or patient documents into recycling bins. Most hospitals will have facilities for **confidential waste** disposal, so ensure that you locate and use these daily.

What is a sharps injury?

A **sharps injury** is when a device such as a needle unintentionally breaks the skin. Various steps can be taken to **minimise** these injuries. Firstly, **immediately dispose** of all sharps. If this is not possible, store them safely in your tray, and ensure that you dispose of your **own** sharps as soon as it is practical – another colleague may be unfamiliar with the number or location of sharps in your tray. However, most clinical settings have **portable sharps bins**, so use them. Common sense dictates that you should **never** try to **remove** anything from a sharps bin, nor should one be **overfilled**. Most have a lockable sliding lid to facilitate closure once full, so that the temptation is minimised to fit 'one more' in.

Never attempt to **re-sheath** a sharp, especially if it has been used.

What should you do if a sharps injury occurs?

Most hospitals have specific **protocols** to follow if a sharps injury occurs. Generally, it is advisable to **encourage bleeding** by squeezing the site. **Wash** the site of injury under **running water** and with **soap**.

Contact **Occupational Health** as soon as possible. They will help with further proceedings – usually involving a **risk assessment** of the 'donor' blood for bloodborne viruses. There are post-exposure prophylactic medications which may be suggested if the risk is **high**. They will usually also arrange for the donor to be actually tested for bloodborne viruses. Do not attempt to approach the patient yourself about this. It is **not acceptable practice** to gain consent for such tests yourself, nor is it acceptable to access their results in this instance – Occupational Health will generally contact you in regard to the results, if appropriate.

Hints and tips:
- Always use **portable sharps** bins if possible.
- Ensure that clinical, domestic and confidential waste matter is disposed of appropriately.
- **Never overfill** or **reach into** a sharps bin.
- **Encourage bleeding** and **wash** a sharps injury.
- **Contact Occupational Health immediately** if you sustain a **sharps injury**.

Did you know?
- Many needles now have **needle safe units** attached to the needle (Figure 3.2). This is usually a **plastic component**, which can click safely and easily over the needle after use – thus minimising the risk of needle-stick injury. If one is present, use it!

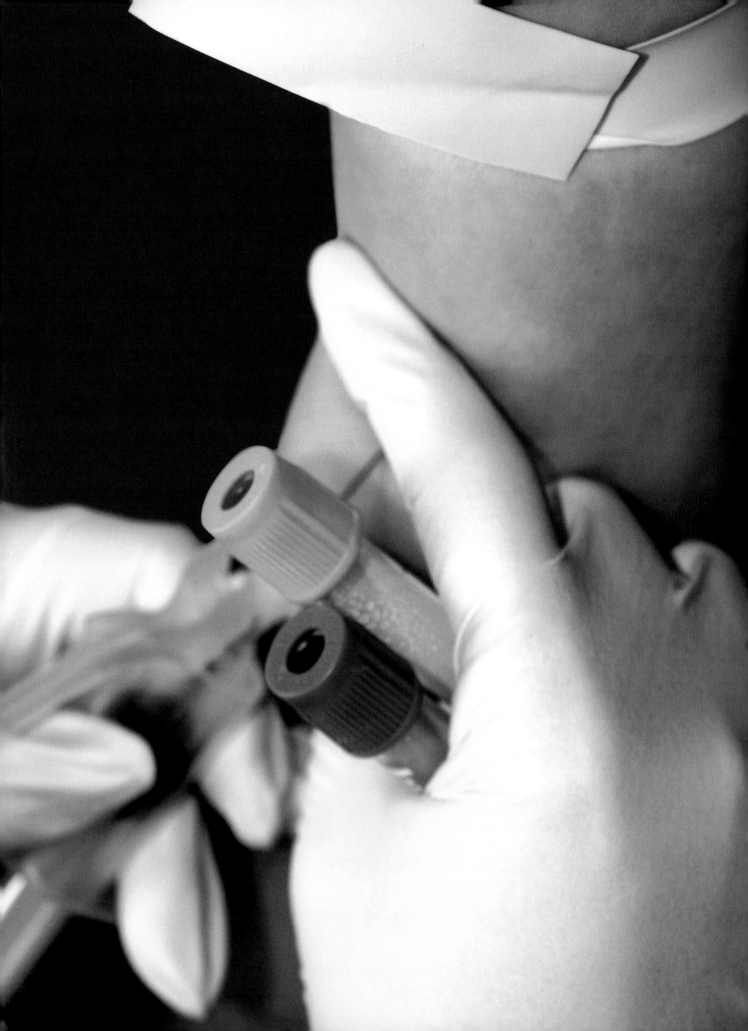

Common preliminary components

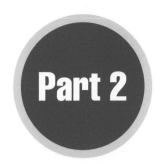

Part 2

Chapters

4 Identifying a patient 10
5 Consent, capacity and documentation 12
6 Hand hygiene and personal protective equipment 14
7 Scrubbing in 16
8 Asepsis 18

4   Identifying a patient

Figure 4.1   Hospital wristbands are important for ID checking

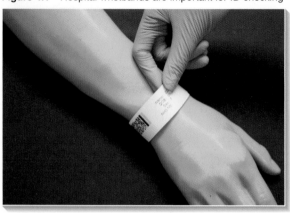

Hints and tips:
- **ID wristbands** must be **present** and **unaltered** on inpatients.
- Ask a patient to state their name, rather than ask: 'Are you….?'
- Perform at least a **two-point** identification on an **alert** patient.
- Perform at least a **three-point** identification on an **unconscious** patient.

Figure 4.2   Use open-ended questions for positive identication

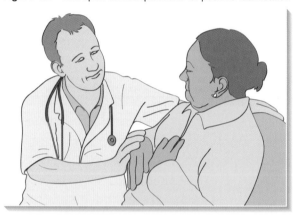

Figure 4.3   Patients must have adhesive ID labels for use in their notes

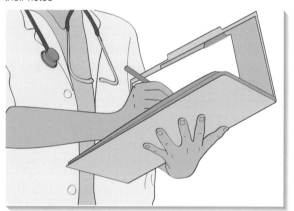

Figure 4.4   The 5 Patient Safety Rights, according to the Department of Health. Source: GS1 Healthcare, GS1 Healthcare Reference Book (2010/2011 ed.), p. 13. Retrieved from http://www.gs1.org/docs/healthcare/GS1_Healthcare_Reference_Book_2010-2011.pdf

1.	Ensuring the right patient
2.	Is given the right treatment
3.	In the right dose
4.	Through the right route
5.	At the right time

Practical Medical Procedures at a Glance, First Edition. Rachel K. Thomas © Rachel K. Thomas. Published 2015 by John Wiley & Sons, Ltd.
Companion website: http://www.ataglanceseries.com/practicalmedprocedures

What is patient identification?

Patient identification is a vitally important aspect of any clinical encounter. It involves checking a patient's information to confirm their identity with multiple pieces of data. It must be **performed correctly**, and the importance of this cannot be stressed enough. Failure to do so results in **harm** to the patient and **penalties** to the Healthcare Trust.

Inpatients must always be wearing **identity wristbands** which are firmly attached and not tampered with, usually on their **dominant arm** (Figure 4.1). This must be secured to the patient after they have been positively identified on admission, and worn throughout their stay in hospital, but its presence does not reduce the responsibility for the medical practitioner to still fully check the patient's identity (Figure 4.2). These wristbands usually contain the patient's **family name**, **given name**, **gender**, **date of birth** and **health system or hospital number**. This amount of information may vary with local protocols. The use of **barcodes** and **quick response (QR) codes** on wristbands is increasing in many hospitals, as they can hold significant amounts of information securely. In some instances, such as with paediatric patients, this band may be secured around the ankle.

Each patient must also have a sheet of **adhesive labels**, containing their relevant information, printed out and included in their medical notes, for use on other pages and documents (Figure 4.3).

Why is identifying a patient important?

Incorrect identification of a patient, and any procedure carried out on the wrong patient, is a **never event**, as decreed by the Department of Health. They publish **best practice guidelines** on identification, and it is the practitioner's responsibility to ensure that these are followed. Any instance where a patient is incorrectly identified may result in **harm** occurring to the patient. The Healthcare Trust where the event occurs, even if there is no serious outcome, is harshly **fined**. Therefore, it is important to prioritise identifying patients correctly early on in your medical training, so that this becomes second nature. While at times it may be tempting to assume a patient's identity for the sake of speed, the few seconds saved can come at a disastrous cost if the identity turns out to be mistaken. Studies have shown that half of all hospital errors are **preventable** – leading to the Department of Health's vision that all patients should have **5 safety rights** – the first of which involves ensuring that the patient is correctly identified (Figure 4.4).

Different types of identification

At the outset of every encounter, a patient needs to be **correctly identified** using **multiple data points** of identification. It is important to use **open-ended questions**, so that the patient provides the information (Figure 4.2). For instance, do not ask, 'Are you Mrs Jones?', as this breaches the confidentiality of the named patient, if the person being questioned is someone else, and may confuse the patient you are attempting to identify. Instead, it is better to ask: "May I please confirm your given and family names?"

A minimum of **two-point identification** is advised for any basic clinical encounter. This requires at least two different sets of information, such as the patient's full name and their date of birth, to be matched against their hospital wristband and notes.

A minimum of **three-point identification** is advised if a patient is **unconscious** or for **invasive procedures** and **blood transfusions**. This involves three sets of information, such as their full name, date of birth and hospital number, to be matched with their wristband and hospital notes.

Requirements for identification may vary according to **local policies**, so be sure to adhere to these.

Aspects of identification

When interacting with a patient, while it is imperative to correctly identify them, it is also important to **introduce** yourself. Ensure that you are wearing **formal identification** such as a medical school name badge or a hospital identification card, and that this can be clearly seen.

Whenever answering a bleep or telephone, it is important to fully identify yourself. Include your **name**, **designation**, **bleep number** and, if possible, usual location or **ward**.

Become familiar with the practices that your workplace adopts if there are patients of the **same name** or of similar names. Some hospitals may use a recognisable **sign** or **symbol** near the patient's bed or on the doctors' ward lists. Some hospitals intentionally place such patients next to each other on the same ward, to reinforce their similar names and thus draw attention to them in efforts to minimise mistakes.

Procedure

The following vocabulary may be appropriate:

"Hello, my name is **Dr Thomas** [gesturing to show formal hospital identification badge], and I am a **junior doctor** on the team that is looking after you here in **Ward 2**."

Ensure that the patient has heard your name and seen your badge, so that they can recall your name if desired.

"May I please confirm your **given name** and your **family name**?"

As the patient replies, **check** their response against the patient **documents** that you have. Request that they spell out the names if required.

"May I please **check** your **wristband**?"

Confirm that the information matches the wristband.

"Please can you confirm your **date of birth**?"

Again, check this against the wristband and the patient documents.

This comprises **two-point identification**, which is the recommended minimum requirement to positively identify them.

It is also advisable to check their hospital number, or address, and these **must** be checked if **three-point identification** is required.

Did you know?

A study carried out in London's Charing Cross Hospital as part of the Department of Health's *Coding for Success* policy revealed that sufficient patient identification checks were performed only 17% of the time. The use of **bar-coded wristbands** improved this to **81%** of the time.

5 Consent, capacity and documentation

Box 5.1 Consent requirements

In order to give **consent**, the patient must:

- Be free from coercion, act **voluntarily**
- Have **capacity**

Box 5.2 Capacity requirements

In order to be deemed as having **capacity**, the patient must be able to:

- **Understand** the information given
- **Retain** the information given
- **Weigh** the information in the balance, considering all aspects and implications of each outcome
- **Communicate** their decision

Figure 5.1 Actions can give implied consent

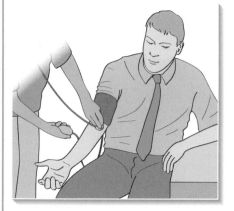

Figure 5.2 A sample of a hospital consent form

Patient identifier/label

Name of proposed procedure or course of treatment (include brief explanation if medical term not clear) ....
....
....

Statement of health professional (to be filled in by health professional with appropriate knowledge of proposed procedure, as specified in consent policy)

I have explained the procedure to the patient. In particular, I have explained:

The intended benefits ....
....
....

Serious or frequently occurring risks ....
....
....

Any extra procedures which may become necessary during the procedure
☐ blood transfusion
☐ other procedure (please specify) ....
....

I have also discussed what the procedure is likely to involve, the benefits and risks of any available alternative treatments (including no treatment) and any particular concerns of this patient.

☐ The following leaflet/tape has been provided ....

This procedure will involve:
☐ general and/or regional anaesthesia   ☐ local anaesthesia   ☐ sedation

Signed: ....   Date: ....
Name (PRINT): ....   Job title: ....

Contact details (if patient wishes to discuss options later) ....

Statement of interpreter (where appropriate)

I have interpreted the information above to the patient to the best of my ability and in a way in which I believe she/he can understand.

Signed: ....   Date: ....
Name (PRINT): ....

Signed: ....

What is consent?

Consent is essentially gaining **permission** from a patient. Gaining consent is required **by law**, **prior to any intervention** – from more simple, non-invasive interventions such as vital sign measurements to complex, invasive procedures such as performing an operation. An **intervention** is basically defined as anything you 'do' to a patient, no matter how small it may seem.

Consent is only valid if it is given **voluntarily**, and if the patient has **capacity at the time** when they are giving it (Box 5.1). Once a patient has given consent, they are still free to **withdraw** this consent, provided that they have the **capacity** to do so, at a later time. Certain areas regarding consent are confusing and difficult, for example areas relating to minors, the refusal of life-saving treatment and the donation of living organs. In these cases, seek **senior expert help**, as some instances may require **High Court decisions**.

Consent can be given in several different ways, with different modes being appropriate for particular interventions. **Words** can convey consent, **actions** can also convey consent and at other times the consent will need to be **formal** and **written**. For example, following a discussion about taking a patient's pulse, a patient then offering their wrist for you to do so may be taken as implied consent (Figure 5.1). Prior to a hip replacement, written informed consent will need to be taken by the surgeon on a formal consent form (Figure 5.2). The intended **risks** and **benefits** of a procedure

Practical Medical Procedures at a Glance, First Edition. Rachel K. Thomas © Rachel K. Thomas. Published 2015 by John Wiley & Sons, Ltd.
Companion website: http://www.ataglanceseries.com/practicalmedprocedures

need to be understood by the patient – and, therefore, do not seek to obtain consent from a patient for a procedure which you are not able to do yourself. The patient also should be informed of **why** an intervention is needed, and **how** it will be carried out if they consent to it.

What is capacity?

Capacity, according to the **Mental Capacity Act 2005**, is the ability to **understand** information, **retain** this information, **weigh** its **outcomes** in the balance and **communicate a decision** (Box 5.2).

Capacity must be present, with all four of these criteria being met, in order for a patient to **legally permit** you to perform any intervention on them. Ensure you document a formal **assessment** of capacity in the patient's notes if there is any question relating to their ability to consent – it does not need to be an excessively long entry, but it does need to convey that the patient is able to:

- **Understand** the information which has been given in regard to the intended intervention.
- **Retain** this information in their mind, on their own.
- **Consider** what the information means, including consideration of both negative and positive outcomes, should the intended intervention occur. They must also be able to consider the negative and positive outcomes that may occur if the intervention does not occur. They must be able to **weigh** these options against each other
- Effectively **communicate** their **decision** after the above requirements have been met. Communication can occur by any effective means.

If a patient has capacity, they are able to **refuse treatment** as well as able to accept it. If you are unsure, it is always better to seek senior help, as treating a patient against their will in such a case constitutes **battery**, a **prosecutable offence**.

Efforts must be made to **optimise** and **enhance** a patient's capacity. If it is lacking, then the patient must be treated in their **best interests**. Senior input should always be sought in these cases, and guidance is also available from resources such as the General Medical Council (GMC). Generally, a patient **over the age of 16** is assumed to **possess capacity** and the ability to consent, unless there is evidence to suggest otherwise. A patient **under the age of 16** is generally presumed to **lack capacity**, unless they can indicate that they are able to understand their condition and the proposed treatments sufficiently. This is regarded to as **Gillick** or **Fraser competence**, named after a landmark case in the House of Lords in 1985. This area can be confusing, and so it is best to seek senior input.

A patient **under the age of 16** who is not deemed Gillick or Fraser competent requires consent from someone with **parental responsibility**. This is usually (but not always) a parent. In emergencies, actions should be carried out in the child's **best interests**. **Court decisions** may need to be applied for in cases where parental responsibility consent cannot be obtained and the child will suffer if the proposed treatments and procedures are not carried out.

Why are consent and capacity important?

Capacity and consent are important for both ethical and legal reasons. They are required in order to **protect** the **patient's rights**,

and they also **protect** the **medical practitioner**. These concepts can, at times, be difficult to evaluate. Therefore, it is always better to ask for **senior help**, as well as assistance from the **Psychiatry** team, the **GMC** and various other resources if you are unsure, as the potentially complicated decisions in this area are beyond those required of a junior medical professional.

What is documentation, and why is it important?

Clear, concise, thorough documentation is a **necessity**.

Documentation involves **recording** various aspects so that they can be referred to at a later date. It includes recording how the patient is, as well as what has been planned and what has occurred. Ensure that you document in the **correct location** – for instance, some hospital protocols require cannula insertion to be documented in the patient's **medication card**. Some hospitals may have **computer** systems for the documentation of thromboembolism risk assessment, whereas others may require this to be completed on **paper**.

Ensure that you always document **neatly** and in **ink**, and remember that patient notes are **legal documents**. Ensure that you use appropriately respectful and formal language, and only acceptable abbreviations. This will facilitate reading of the notes by other professionals involved in the patient's care.

Be sure to document any **attempts** at procedures, even if they are unsuccessful. If something is **not documented**, it is assumed to have **not happened**. Do not be embarrassed or feel the need to hide any failed attempts.

If you have attempted to contact another team for a **referral**, include this in the patient notes – including who you spoke to, their bleep number or contact details and when they agreed to review your patient.

Thorough documentation is imperative for good clinical care. It will also help you to protect yourself against, and to deal with, any future questions or **complaints**, so ensure that you document neatly and fully at all times. Inquiries and complaints can arise **years** after contact, so be as thorough as possible. While it is obvious that no one likes to be complained about, complaints can provide **useful feedback** to assist you in developing as a communicator and a clinician. It may be that the complaint was directed at you but actually made for other reasons (e.g. frustration at an ineffective treatment or a sense of loss from a bereavement), and it may still help inform your future practice. Complaints must be dealt with **honestly** and **openly**. It may be advisable to seek input from a **medical defence union** or a **senior** if you are unsure how best to proceed.

Hints and tips:
- Seek **senior help** if you are unsure as to a patient's ability to consent.
- **Good communication skills** facilitate gaining consent – ensure **appropriate language** is used.
- Ensure patients understand they can later **withdraw** their consent, if they have capacity at that time.
- **Never** obtain consent for procedures which you **cannot perform** yourself.

6 Hand hygiene and personal protective equipment

Figure 6.1 Six steps for adequate handwashing

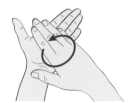

1. Rub palm to palm

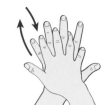

2. Rub the back of both hands

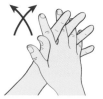

3. Rub palm to palm interlacing the fingers

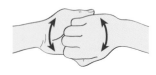

4. Rub the backs of fingers by interlocking the hands

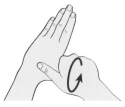

5. Rub the thumbs

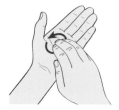

6. Rub palms with fingertips

Figure 6.2 Standard practice: the 5 moments of hand hygiene. Source: Sax *et al* (2007), Figure 2. Reproduced with permission of Elsevier.

1.	**Before patient contact**	*When?*	Clean your hands before touching a patient when approaching him or her
		Why?	To protect the patient against harmful germs carried on your hands
2.	**Before an aseptic task**	*When?*	Clean your hands immediately before any aseptic task
		Why?	To protect the patient against harmful germs, including the patient's own germs, entering his or her body
3.	**After body fluid exposure risk**	*When?*	Clean your hands immediately after an exposure risk to body fluids (and after glove removal)
		Why?	To protect yourself and the health-care environment from harmful patient germs
4.	**After patient contact**	*When?*	Clean your hands after touching a patient and his or her immediate surroundings when leaving
		Why?	To protect yourself and the health-care environment from harmful patient germs
5.	**After contact with patient surroundings**	*When?*	Clean your hands after touching any object or furniture in the patient's immediate surrondings, when leaving - even without touching the patient
		Why?	To protect yourself and the health-care environment from harmful patient germs

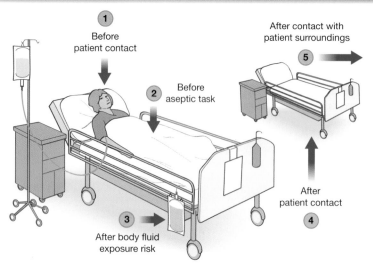

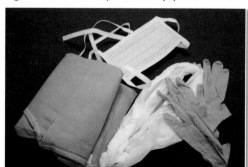

Figure 6.3 Personal protective equipment

Source: World Health Organization (2009). Reproduced with permission of World Health Organization.

Practical Medical Procedures at a Glance, First Edition. Rachel K. Thomas © Rachel K. Thomas. Published 2015 by John Wiley & Sons, Ltd.
Companion website: http://www.ataglanceseries.com/practicalmedprocedures

What is hand hygiene?

Hand hygiene involves adequately **cleaning** the hands and lower arms at various points of interaction with patients. It is a **World Health Organization (WHO)** directive. Good hand hygiene behaviour **decreases** the **microbe load** and breaks the chain of infection, rather than creating a sterile environment.

Alcoholic gels and **rubs** are often present in hospitals – these are adequate for **basic hygiene**, but a thorough handwashing with water and an antibacterial agent or soap needs to be performed prior to invasive procedures and after interacting with patients with loose stools. Thorough handwashing occurs in **six steps** (Figure 6.1). This should occur at five moments (Figure 6.2). These six steps should be utilised if the hands are being cleaned with a gel or rub, or with water and soap or an antibacterial agent.

Most Healthcare Trusts have a '**bare below the elbows**' policy. This requires that healthcare professionals ensure they have no articles of clothing or items such as watches or bracelets on their lower arms. (In some Healthcare Trusts, a single, simple wedding band may be worn.) This facilitates handwashing – more effective handwashing occurs when the cleaning of the wrist is not impeded by watches and sleeves – rather than improving infection control. Therefore, shirts must be short sleeved or have the sleeves rolled up to above the elbow, and watches must be removed.

Equipment such as stethoscopes should be regularly disinfected by use of alcohol wipes or soap and water.

A more extensive 'scrubbing in' process is used prior to admission for surgical procedures, but the basic steps are essentially the same. In this situation, the process is repeated 3–5 times depending on the preparation used (see Chapter 7).

> **Did you know?**
>
> The **six steps** for handwashing were determined by Ayliffe *et al.* (1978) in tests for 'hygienic' hand disinfection, and they are now **standard practice**.

What is personal protective equipment?

Personal protective equipment (PPE) includes various items used to decrease personal exposure to infection. These items include **disposable gloves, masks, goggles, hair caps, gowns, aprons** and **shoe covers**. The following is not an exhaustive list of indications for the use of PPE, and both common sense and hospital protocols dictate their use (Figure 6.3).

Non-sterile, disposable, single-use gloves should be worn whenever touching **contaminated** or **infectious materials** such as blood or body substances, or when touching patient areas such as mucous membranes, broken skin or internal areas. They should also be used to protect the medical practitioner from **potentially dangerous substances**, according to Health and Safety requirements such as the **Control of Substances Hazardous to Health (COSHH)**.

Hand hygiene steps should be performed **prior** to putting on the gloves, and immediately **after** their removal. Evidence suggests that microbes and bacteria flourish in the 'greenhouse' that the gloves may create whilst they are on, and that hands are contaminated when the gloves are removed.

Gloves should be changed during a procedure if they are visibly **soiled** or **torn**, and between **different procedures** on the same patient. They must be changed after contact with **each patient**. They do not replace the need for the six steps of hand hygiene,

at the five moments of clinical interaction, nor do they protect against needle-stick or other sharps injuries (see Chapter 3).

Sterile, disposable, single-use gloves must be worn for any procedure that requires **aseptic techniques** (see Chapter 8).

Masks and **goggles** should be worn to protect from procedures where there is the possibility of **body fluids splashing** into the eyes, nose or mouth of the practitioner. Ventilation masks should also be used in situations where patients require ventilation, rather than directly proceeding to 'mouth-to-mouth' procedures.

Hair caps should be used in theatre, or for appropriate procedures on the wards, and hair should always be neat and tied back if it is longer than shoulder length.

Gowns and **aprons** should be worn to protect skin and clothing in procedures both in theatre and on the wards.

Why are hand hygiene and PPE important?

Hands are the most common vehicles for **transmitting infection** between patients. Therefore, handwashing is the most important measure for **controlling infection**, as adequate hand cleaning helps break the transmission cycle.

PPE is of **double-fold** value, protecting both the practitioner and the patient from the spread of microorganisms and infection.

Procedure

Handwashing can be done with alcoholic rubs, or with medicated soaps and antibacterial agents.

These **six steps** should be performed prior to every point of patient contact, and after every point of patient contact. It is standard practice for this to be performed at the **five moments** (Figure 6.2):

1 Ensure **bare below the elbows**, by rolling up sleeves, or removing long-sleeved clothing if appropriate, and removing watches, bracelets and rings (according to local hospital protocols – some may permit a single plain wedding band. If so, be sure to slide it up and down the digit to facilitate cleaning the skin underneath it).
2 **Introduce** yourself, and **identify** the patient (see Chapter 4).
3 Gain **consent** for the procedure (see Chapter 5), explain **indications** and check for **contra-indications** or **allergies**.
4 **Don apron**, and a **mask** if required.
5 **Wash hands** using the **six steps** of hand hygiene (Figure 6.1):
  a Rub both of the palms together.
  b Rub the back of each hand with the palm of the other hand.
  c Rub the palms together while interlacing the fingers.
  d Rub the backs of the fingers with the other hand's palm, while interlocking the fingers.
  e Rub the thumb by wrapping and rotating the other hand around it.
  f Rub the fingertips into the other hand's palm.
6 **Dry** the hands using a clean disposable towel.

Repeat at the **five moments** of a clinical encounter, or as clinically appropriate.

> **Hints and tips:**
>
> • Remember – **alcoholic rubs** are not effective against some bacteria, such as *Clostridium difficile*.
> • Ensure PPE waste is disposed of in the **appropriate** containers – it is **clinical waste**.
> • Ensure hands are washed both **immediately before** donning gloves, and **immediately after** their removal.

7 Scrubbing in

Figure 7.1   Sterile surgical gown pack

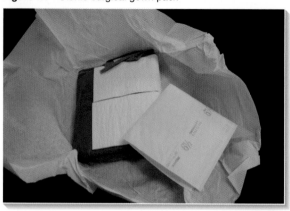

Hints and tips:
- **Prepare** all your equipment.
- Remember your **glove size**.
- Ensure hands are **thoroughly** dry prior to **donning gloves** – or else they seem **sticky**!
- **Scrub nurses** are usually happy to help.
- **Start again** if there is a possibility that you have **desterilised** yourself.

Figure 7.2   (a, b) Donning sterile gloves

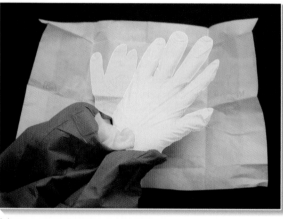

(a)

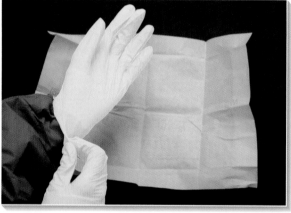

(b)

Figure 7.3   Scrubbed in for theatre

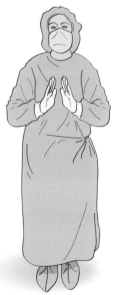

Did you know?

There are two main types of handwashing solution:
1. **Iodine based**, which is **brown** in colour
2. **Chlorhexidine based**, which is **pink** in colour

Both are usually available, so use whichever you prefer.

Practical Medical Procedures at a Glance, First Edition. Rachel K. Thomas © Rachel K. Thomas. Published 2015 by John Wiley & Sons, Ltd.
Companion website: http://www.ataglanceseries.com/practicalmedprocedures

What is scrubbing in?

Scrubbing in, also known as **surgical scrubbing** or **scrubbing up**, is a necessary step for involvement in **theatre**, and for other **invasive procedures**. It involves several steps, none of which are complicated, such as donning personal protective equipment and thoroughly washing the hands (see Chapter 6). The aim is to provide a **sterile surface**, consisting of a gown and gloves, through which you can interact with the patient and perform or assist in an aseptic procedure.

Why is scrubbing in important?

Scrubbing in is an important **infection control procedure**, and is thus needed to provide **good clinical care**. It is a prerequisite for involvement in **theatre**, and accordingly, is a skill best mastered early on. While its steps may seem easy, it is important to perform them correctly. Any accidents along the way, leading to **contamination** and **de-sterilisation**, require starting the process again. It is imperative to admit when you have inadvertently de-sterilised yourself, no matter how trivial you think it may be at the time. By having to begin the scrubbing-in process again, you are at worst slightly delaying the theatre start time. This is far preferable to **knowingly adding infection** to a surgical wound, leading to potentially **disastrous consequences** for the patient.

Aspects of scrubbing in

Prior to beginning the handwashing, ensure that you have all equipment ready. **Preparation** is the key! Many Healthcare Trusts store **hair caps** in their change rooms. When you are putting on your **scrubs** and **theatre shoes**, remember to collect and don a hair cap at this time. **Face masks** and **face shields** are PPE (see Chapter 6) which are often stored in theatre – these may include a thin plastic visor to protect your eyes. If you wear glasses, these usually suffice. Ensure that you tie the mask securely but comfortably, and adjust the metal strip inside the nose bridge for comfort if it is present. After this point, you will need to ask a colleague to readjust it for you, as it is not sterile and therefore cannot be touched once you commence scrubbing in. According to local protocols, a **scrub sponge** and **nail-cleaning tool** may be required for the first scrub of the day.

Sterile gowns and **sterile gloves** are **pre-packed** and stored in theatre (Figure 7.1). Prior to handwashing, the gown pack will need to be opened onto a clean surface, and its internal packaging unwrapped by pulling only at the corners. This will provide a **sterile field**, containing the folded gown. Decide on your glove size, and remember this. These will need to be opened and **dropped** into the sterile field, being sure not to touch anything. For donning the gown when you have washed your hands, hold its top edges near the necktie, and let it gently roll and unfold open, being careful to not let it touch anything. Wriggle your hands into the sleeves, but do not let the hands protrude from the ends. Use your hands in **pincer movements**, as though in mittens, inside the ends of the sleeves to manipulate on the gloves (Figure 7.2a). This takes practice and time, so try to avoid feeling rushed the first few times you attempt it. Once your hand is partially inside the glove, its cuff can be pulled down and the hand fully inserted. Donning the first glove is the most difficult, as once one hand is gloved, it can be used to assist in the gloving of the other (Figure 7.2b).

Once fully scrubbed in, move around the theatre **carefully**, and with **arms crossed** or **palms together**, to decrease the risk of contaminating yourself.

Procedure

Change into **theatre scrubs** (shirt and trousers) and **theatre shoes** in the change room.

- **Don hair cap**.
- **Don face mask**.
- **Open** the **surgical gown pack** onto a clean surface, and gently pull the corners of the inner wrapping paper diagonally apart.
- **Open sterile gloves**, and drop them into the sterile field of the gown pack without touching anything in the field.
- **Open scrub sponge** if one is required in the Healthcare Trust policy.
- Turn on water, and dispense **disinfectant** or **antibacterial agent** using your elbows.
- **Wash hands** (see Chapter 6) (use the scrub sponge to clean more thoroughly, if required).
- Rinse your hands by holding them **vertically** under the flowing water, so that it runs from your fingertips to mid-forearm.
- Repeat **3–5 times**, as per local protocol.
- Turn off the taps with your **elbows**.
- **Dry hands** with **sterile towels** – using one per hand.
- **Don gown** by inserting hands into each sleeve.
- **Don gloves,** ensuring that your skin does not touch the exterior of the gloves or the gown.
- **Secure gown** with assistance of a colleague (Figure 7.3).

8 Asepsis

Figure 8.1 Key parts which must not be touched

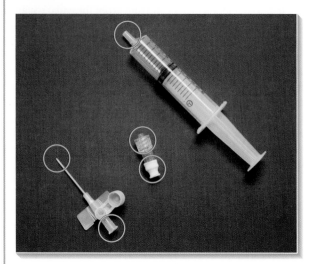

Figure 8.2 Key parts can be protected by careful insertion back into their original packaging

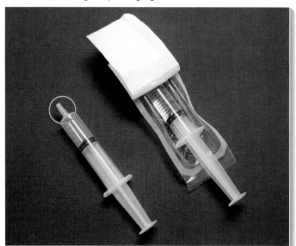

Figure 8.3 Example of a sterile dressing pack once opened

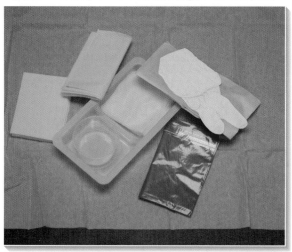

Hints and tips:

- Always perform the **six steps of handwashing** (see Chapter 6).
- Wash hands **before** and **after** donning sterile gloves,
- Try not to obsessively apply hand gel, but consider the **five moments of hand hygiene** (see Chapter 6).

Box 8.1 Aseptic non-touch technique (ANTT). Adapted from www.antt.org

	The 10 principles:
1.	The **Medical Practitioner** is the **main infection risk** to the patient during a procedure.
2.	**Asepsis** is the **infection prevention** aim of all invasive clinical procedures. **Medical Practitioners** must **establish** and **maintain** it.
3.	It is **vital** to **identify** and **protect key parts** and **key sites**
4.	**ANTT** is used to maintain asepsis for **all clinical procedures**.
5.	The technical difficulty of the procedure should be **risk assessed**.
6.	**Aseptic fields** are important – these fields may be managed with standard or surgical ANTT.
7.	The most important component of ANTT is the **non-touch technique**.
8.	Asepsis is promoted and ensured by appropriate anti-infective precautions.
9.	There should be **standard use** of **aseptic practice**.
10.	Appropriate staff training, environments and equipment are needed for safe **aseptic technique**.

Practical Medical Procedures at a Glance, First Edition. Rachel K. Thomas © Rachel K. Thomas. Published 2015 by John Wiley & Sons, Ltd.
Companion website: http://www.ataglanceseries.com/practicalmedprocedures

What is aseptic technique?

Aseptic technique (also called the **aseptic non-touch technique**, or **ANTT**) is a method frequently used in medical practice that involves **minimising** the possibility of **infectious contamination** (Box 8.1). It is used as the **basic pre-procedure** before procedures such as wound care, bladder catheterisation and chest drain insertion. It involves identifying **key sites** and **key parts**, and then adhering to the underlying principles of **ANTT**:

- Always **wash hands** effectively.
- Never contaminate **key parts**.
- Touch **non-key parts** with confidence.
- Take appropriate anti-infective **precautions**.

Key sites are sites in the body through which **infection may be introduced** during a procedure. These include open wounds, insertion sites such as the urethral meatus and puncture sites such as in phlebotomy or cannulation.

Key parts (Figure 8.1) are the parts of the equipment you are using that, if contaminated, may **introduce infection into the key sites**. For example, key parts include the following (although there are many more examples):

- Catheter tip, end or drainage bag connector
- Needle-free bung
- Syringe
- Saline flush top
- Cannula and port
- Infusion set ports
- Culture bottle tops

In carrying out ANTT, it is very important to **identify key sites** and **key parts**, and to ensure that these remain **uncontaminated**. **Key parts should only come into contact with key sites** – not with your fingers or any other potentially contaminated surface. To help prevent contamination, when preparing an equipment tray, key parts can be stored back inside their **original package** to maintain sterility (Figure 8.2).

Why do it?

Aseptic technique is a simple but **incredibly important skill** for all healthcare professionals to master. Good technique will help to minimise the number of **healthcare-associated infections (HCAIs)**.

> **Did you know?**
>
> **HCAIs** (or **nosocomial infections**) are infections that patients contract *in hospital* or in a *healthcare setting* – often as a result of **poor aseptic technique**. Those infections responsible for the most morbidity and mortality are methicillin-resistant *Staphylococcus aureus* (MRSA) and *Clostridium difficile* gastroenteritis.

Procedure

- **Introduce** yourself, and **identify** the patient (see Chapter 4).
- Gain **consent** for the procedure (see Chapter 5), explain **indications** and check for **contra-indications** or **allergies**.

- Ensure **bare below the elbows**, and **wash hands** (see Chapter 6).
- Put on an **apron**.
- **Clean trolley** with a chlorhexadine wipe.
- Gather equipment, and put it on the lower shelf of the trolley.
- **Wash hands** with alcohol gel or soap.
- **Open wound-dressing pack** (Figure 8.3) onto the clean surface of the trolley, being careful not to touch any of the sterile contents. To open carefully, **hold the corners** of the pack. Do not touch anywhere else.
- Place any other equipment you need by opening their packets and **dropping** them directly onto the **sterile field** you have created with the dressing pack.
- Open a pair of **sterile gloves**.
- **Wash hands** and don the **sterile gloves**. Clean and dress the patient's wound appropriately.
- Dispose of contaminated equipment and packaging in appropriate clinical waste bins, including gloves.
- **Wash hands**.
- Clean trolley.

Aspects of ANTT

Sometimes, it is necessary to use **surgical ANTT** rather than standard or **non-surgical ANTT**. This is usually the case when the procedure is **prolonged** and more **complex** and there are a **larger number** of **key sites** and **key parts**. The differences between the two are summarised in Table 8.1.

Table 8.1 Comparison of standard and surgical ANTT

Procedure	Standard	Surgical
Handwashing	Six steps at five moments, using alcohol gel or soap	Scrubbing in
Protective personal equipment	Apron	Surgical gown
Gloves	May be sterile	Always sterile
Surfaces	Disinfected trolley	Sterile drapes used

In some cases, it may be appropriate to take **swabs** of wounds. These should be taken using a **sterile wound swab**. After gently gaining a sample by moving the swab over the wound while rotating it, the swab is placed in its transport tube's carrier medium, labelled and sent to **Microbiology** along with the appropriate request form. Ensure that the swab tip only touches the area to be tested. Swabs are commonly taken of the skin, and areas such as the nose and throat, in order to help determine the presence of **infective organisms** and their **antibiotic sensitivities**.

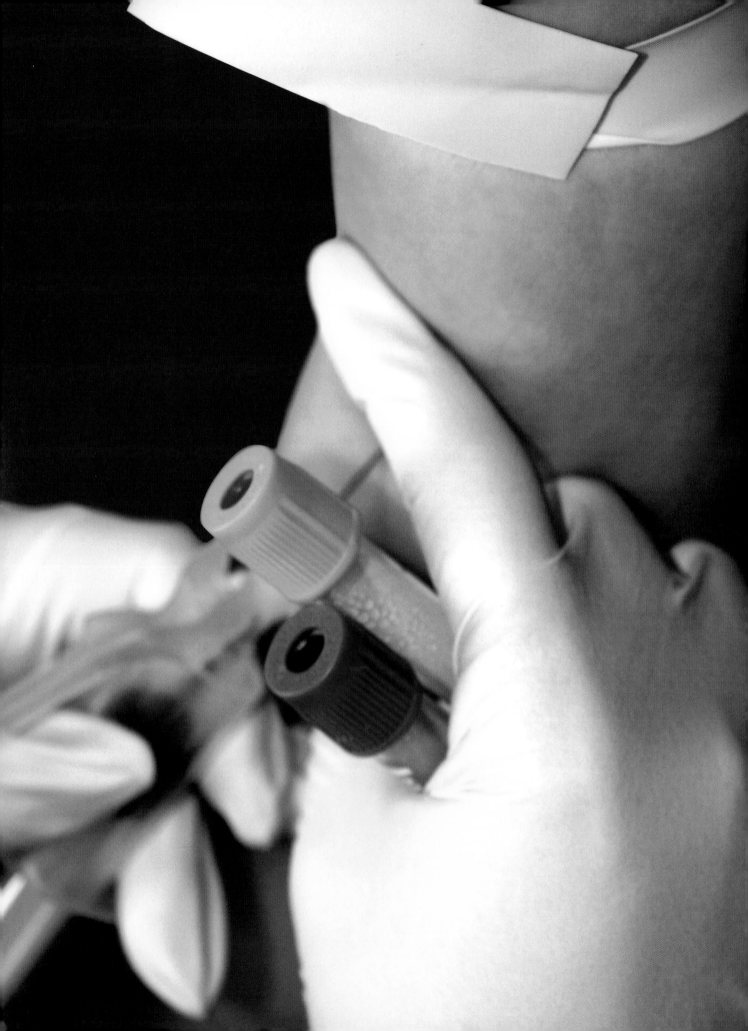

Common non-invasive ward procedures

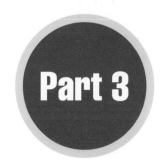

Part 3

Chapters

9   Measuring vital signs   22
10   Writing a safe prescription   24

9 Measuring vital signs

Figure 9.1 A typical trolley for taking measurements

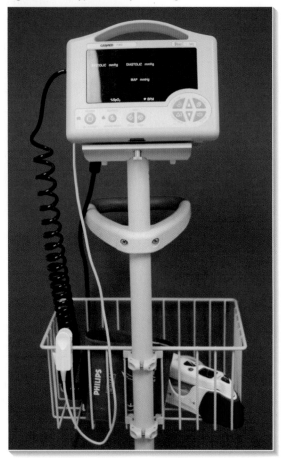

Figure 9.2 Vital signs recorded on an observation chart

Hospital Observation record					
Date		2/10	2/10	2/10	2/10
Time		0800	1200	1600	2000
SpO₂	O₂ therapy		N/C	N/C	
	O₂ L/min	R/A	2	2	
	SpO₂	95	94	94	
Respiratory rate	>30 Score 3				
	21–29 Score 2			21	
	15–20 Score 1		16		
	9–14 Score 0	14			
	Score 1				
	<9 Score 2				
	7 or below Score 3				
	Resp score	0	1	2	
Temperature	Score 3				
	>38.5 Score 2			38.6	
	Score 1				
	35–38.4 Score 0	38.2	38.4		
	Score 1				
	<35 Score 2				
	Score 3				
	Temp score	0	0	2	
AVPU	A Score 0	A	A	A	
	V Score 1				
	Score 2				
	P, U Score 3				
	AVPU score	0	0	0	
Heart rate	<40 Score 2 200				
	41–50 Score 1 190				
	51–100 Score 0 180				
	101–110 Score 1 170				
	111–129 Score 2 160				
	>130 Score 3 150				
	140				
	130				
	120				
	110				
	100				
Systolic blood pressure	<70 Score 3 90				
	71–80 Score 2 80				
	81–100 Score 1 70				
	101–199 Score 0 60				
	Score 1 50				
	>200 Score 2 40				
	HR score	0	0	1	
	Sys BP score	0	0	0	
	TOTAL SCORE	0	1	5	
	Escalated?	Y/N	Y/N	Y/N	Y/N
	Initials	AD	AD	AD	

Table 9.1 MEWS – modified early warning system. Source: Subbe *et al* (2001). Reproduced with permission of Oxford University Press.

Score	3	2	1	0	1	2	3
Systolic BP	<70	71–80	81–100	101–199		≥200	
Heart rate (bpm)		40	41–50	51–100	101–110	111–129	≥130
Respiratory rate (bpm)		<9		9–14	15–20	21–29	>30
Temperature (°C)		<35		35.0–38.4		≥38.5	
AVPU score				Alert	Reacting to voice	Reacting to pain	Unresponsive

Hints and tips:

- If the patient is **peripherally shut down** or is wearing **nail varnish**, oxygen saturation probe readings at the fingertip may be inaccurate – consider using an earlobe instead.
- **Manually check** any automated device **blood pressure** reading which seems at odds with the clinical picture of the patient.
- Feeling the pulse both **centrally** and **peripherally** can help in determining irregular heartbeats, such as in atrial fibrillation.

Figure 9.3 Oxygen saturation probe

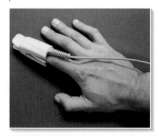

Figure 9.4 Manually recording blood pressure

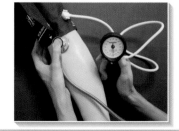

Figure 9.5 (a, b) Tympanic recording of temperature

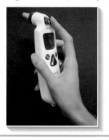
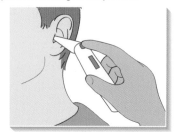

Practical Medical Procedures at a Glance, First Edition. Rachel K. Thomas © Rachel K. Thomas. Published 2015 by John Wiley & Sons, Ltd.
Companion website: http://www.ataglanceseries.com/practicalmedprocedures

What are vital signs?

Vital signs are **measurements** of a patient taken to indicate their **clinical state**. The five vital signs that are commonly recorded are:

- **Respiratory rate**
- **Heart rate**
- **Blood pressure**
- **Temperature**
- **Oxygen saturation**.

They are often measured by nursing staff, and they should be measured and recorded for every patient with **varying clinically appropriate frequencies**. Equipment for measuring the vital signs is commonly on a **trolley** on the ward (Figure 9.1).

Why are vital signs important?

The **vital signs** are taken and recorded to show both **absolute values** and **clinical trends**. These trends can help to provide an early indication of whether a patient is improving or deteriorating, or whether a therapy is effective. They are commonly recorded on **patient observation charts** (Figure 9.2).

Many **Healthcare Trust** protocols have a type of **early warning trigger system**, whereby extremely abnormal values or a combination of mildly abnormal values require immediate action (Table 9.1). Familiarise yourself with these protocols, if they are present.

Procedure

- **Introduce** yourself, and **identify** the patient (see Chapter 4).
- Gain **consent** for the procedure (see Chapter 5), explain **indications** and check for **contra-indications** or **allergies**.
- Ensure **bare below the elbows**, and **wash hands** (see Chapter 6). (Apparatus for collecting information can be attached in any order, as appropriate for the **clinical situation**, and they are specified in no particular order as follows.)
- **Oxygen saturation**: attach **oxygen saturation probe** onto either the patient's **finger** or **earlobe** (Figure 9.3), ensuring that the **inhaled oxygen concentration** is noted and **recorded** as this is needed to give context to the values.
- **Respiratory rate**: **time** for **30 seconds**, and **count** the number of breaths inhaled during this period. **Multiply** this number by two to obtain the respiratory rate in minutes. The respirations can be **seen** on close inspection of the patient's chest, or by **auscultation** with a stethoscope (this is particularly appropriate with paediatric and unwell patients, due to their elevated respiratory rates).
- **Blood pressure**: attach the **deflated blood pressure cuff** to the patient's arm, ensuring that the inflatable bladder is positioned correctly as per the design (it will usually have a mark indicating where the artery below should lie) and that the correctly sized cuff is fitted **snugly** (Figure 9.4). Blood pressure may be measured using an **automatic device**, which will inflate the cuff and give both systolic and diastolic values. It is not advisable to rely solely on these automated readings, particularly in cases where the result differs from what is expected from the clinical picture.

To **manually** determine the blood pressure, **inflate the cuff** by squeezing the pump of the **sphygmomanometer** whilst **palpating** either the radial or brachial pulse until no pulsations can be felt – this is an **estimate** of the **systolic value**. Palpate the artery whilst **deflating the cuff**, *then* place the stethoscope on the brachial artery and **re-inflate the cuff** by squeezing the pump until **no arterial pulsations** can be heard. **Slowly deflate the cuff**, watching the **pressure gauge** and **listening** carefully over the artery. Note the value at which the pulsations are **heard** again – this is the **systolic pressure value**, with the pulsations heard being caused

by turbulent arterial flow. **Continue deflating the cuff** until the pulsations **muffle** or are **not heard** – this is the **diastolic pressure value**, with the muffling or disappearance of the pulsations due to the flow becoming smoother and more laminar again. The estimations with palpation should always be performed in order to **avoid underestimating** the **systolic pressure**, which can occur if only auscultation is used. Record as the **systolic pressure value/diastolic pressure value**. In some clinical indications, it may be relevant to record this with the patient supine, and then standing.

- **Pulse rate**: **time** for **30 seconds**, **palpate** and **count** a **distal pulse** (commonly the radial pulse) and **multiply** this by two to obtain the pulse rate in minutes. Assess if it is **regular** or **irregular**. It may also be assessed by **auscultation** of the praecordium (chest).
- **Temperature**: this can be recorded with various devices. **Tympanic thermometers** are the most common, and their use varies slightly according to each type of device (Figure 9.5a and 9.5b). Generally, place a new plastic sleeve over the device sensor, and **insert** into the patient's ear, angling the sensor forward and down. **Press** the activation button, generally until a bleep is heard and a value is displayed on the screen. (Other methods for measuring a temperature include axillary, rectal and sublingual measurements with sterile thermometers.)
- **Record each value** in the **patient notes**. Depending on hospital protocols, these values may also need to be recorded on the **patient's observation chart** (Figure 9.2).
- **Dispose of waste**, such as plastic covers from tympanic thermometers.
- Thank the patient, and ensure they are comfortable and are suffering no adverse effects.
- **Wash hands**.
- **Observe trends** as well as the **absolute values** of each vital sign.
- **Calculate a Modified Early Warning System (MEWS)** score or **early warning values**, and take further actions as required by absolute values, trends or local protocols (Table 9.1).

Aspects of vital signs

The vital signs results that are obtained need to be acted upon promptly. It is key that both the **absolute values** of the results are considered, as well as the **trend** that they are presenting.

An **elevated respiratory rate** is an accurate and **early sign** of an unwell or deteriorating patient, and it should not be ignored. An **elevated temperature** may signify the need for a 'septic screen' in many hospital protocols, including but not limited to chest and abdominal X-rays, swabs (see Chapter 8), blood tests (see Chapter 11), blood cultures (see Chapter 12), urine dipstick (see Chapter 30) and an electrocardiogram (see Chapter 26).

It is key that the results are **recorded** both in the patient's notes and on the patient's observation chart. Recording them immediately on the patient's chart enables trends to be identified early and accurately – enabling appropriate treatments to be both **instigated** and **monitored**.

Did you know?

- Blood pressure is measured **indirectly** with the cuff, using **Korotkoff sounds**, named after a Russian physician who discovered them in 1905. The **1st Korotkoff sound** (when sounds are heard) indicates the **systolic pressure**. The **5th Korotkoff sound** (when sounds disappear) indicates the **diastolic pressure**. If the sounds do not disappear, the **4th Korotkoff sound** (when sounds first muffle) indicates the **diastolic pressure**.
- Blood pressure can also be measured **directly**, using an intra-arterial catheter, usually on unwell patients.

Writing a safe prescription

Figure 10.1 Patient information and allergies section of medication card

A Hospital Medication and Administration Record

Date of Admission	2 / 10 / 20 15
Date of Planned Discharge	8 / 10 / 20 15

Discharge Written	Discharge Destination	Discharge Screened
Initials Date	Initials Date	Initials Date

Patient requires Monitored Dose System for Discharge
Not required ✓   New ☐   Established ☐

Chart Number 1 of 1

Name (surname): JONES	Hospital number: 335297	Consultant: PETERS
First names: HENRY	Date of birth: 10/10/79	Ward: KING
Height 192 cm	Weight 90 kg	Site: Bed 2
Signature: R. Thomas		Date: 2/10/15

Hypersensitivities & Allergies

Hypersensitivities

Agent	Details	Signature	Date
PENICILLIN	**ANAPHYLAXIS**	R. Thomas	2/10/15
ASPIRIN	SKIN RASH	R. Thomas	2/10/15

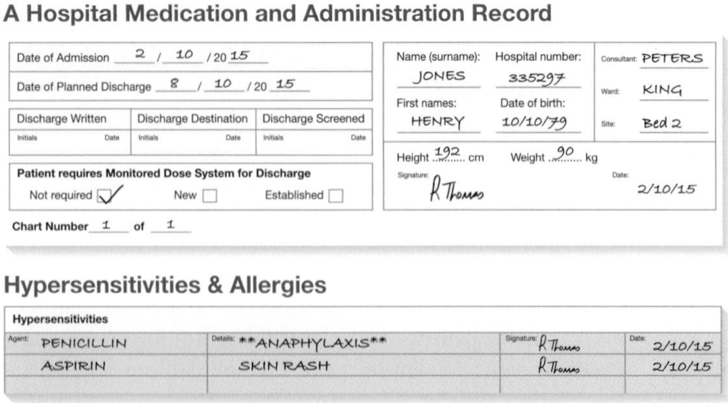

Figure 10.2 Regular medications section of medication card

Regular Medications

Month & Year OCTOBER 2015 Date		2	3	4	5	6	
Medication METRONIDAZOLE	Start date 2/10/15				R/N		
Dose 400mg Route PO Frequency TDS Pharmacy	0800	JR	RS	KL			
Duration, indication 5/7, GI INFECTION	1400	JR	KL	KL			
Signature R. Thomas Print Name RACHEL THOMAS Bleep #426	2200	WP	RS				
Medication PARACETAMOL	Start date 2/10/15				R/N		
Dose 1g Route PO Frequency QDS Pharmacy	0800	AD	AD	KL			
Duration, indication 5/7, PAIN	1400	LP	JP	KL			
Signature R. Thomas Print Name RACHEL THOMAS Bleep #426	1800	LP	JP	KL			
	2200	LP	KL				
Medication	Start date						
Dose Route Frequency Pharmacy							
Duration, indication							

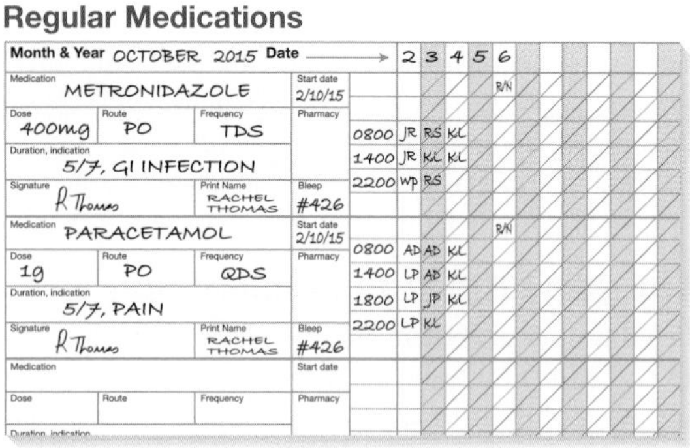

Figure 10.3 'Once only medications' section of medication card

Once Only Medications

Date	Time	Medication	Dose	Route	Signature	Given			Pharmacy
						Date	Time	Initials	
2/10/15	1400	ORAMORPH	5ml	PO	R. Thomas	2/10/15	1410	AK	ML

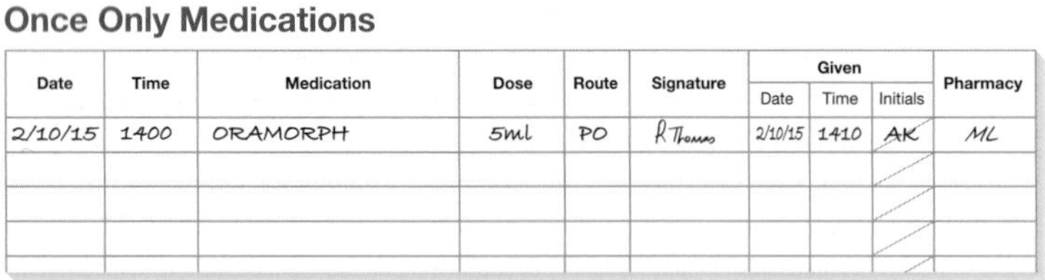

Figure 10.4 'When required medications' section of medication card

When Required Medications

Medication LACTULOSE	Start date 2/10/15	Date	2	4			
Dose 15ml Route PO Frequency PRN/BD Pharmacy		Time	1500	1400			
Indication CONSTIPATION		Dose	15ml	15ml			
		Route	PO	PO			
Signature R. Thomas Print Name RACHEL THOMAS Bleep #426		Given by	AS	KL			
Medication	Start date	Date					
Dose Route Frequency Pharmacy		Time					
Duration, indication		Dose					
		Route					
Signature Print Name Bleep		Given by					
Medication	Start date	Date					
Dose Route Frequency Pharmacy		Time					
Indication		Dose					

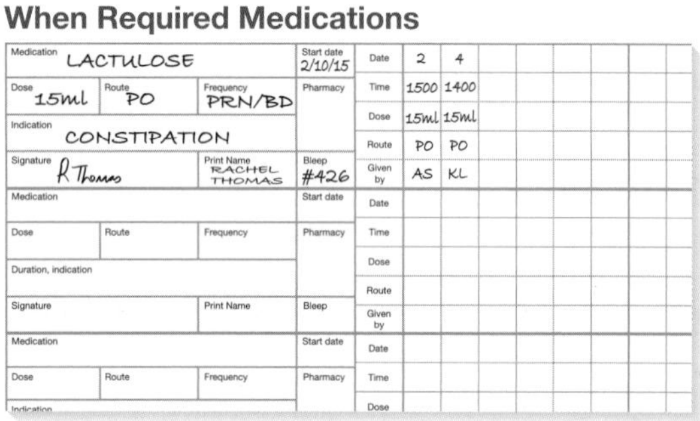

Figure 10.5 'Yellow Card' notification for suspected adverse drug reactions. Source: Yellow Card reporting form. Reproduced with permission from the Medicines and Healthcare Products Regulatory Agency (MHRA).

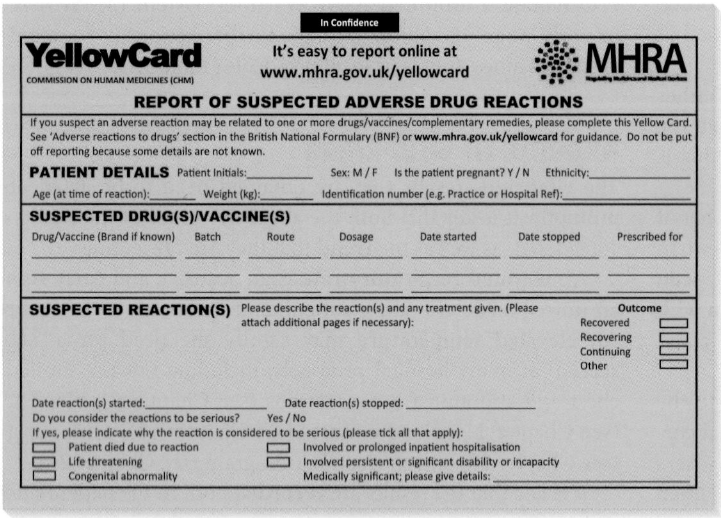

In Confidence

YellowCard
COMMISSION ON HUMAN MEDICINES (CHM)

It's easy to report online at
www.mhra.gov.uk/yellowcard

MHRA

REPORT OF SUSPECTED ADVERSE DRUG REACTIONS

If you suspect an adverse reaction may be related to one or more drugs/vaccines/complementary remedies, please complete this Yellow Card. See 'Adverse reactions to drugs' section in the British National Formulary (BNF) or www.mhra.gov.uk/yellowcard for guidance. Do not be put off reporting because some details are not known.

PATIENT DETAILS Patient Initials: _____ Sex: M / F Is the patient pregnant? Y / N Ethnicity: _____
Age (at time of reaction): _____ Weight (kg): _____ Identification number (e.g. Practice or Hospital Ref): _____

SUSPECTED DRUG(S)/VACCINE(S)

Drug/Vaccine (Brand if known)	Batch	Route	Dosage	Date started	Date stopped	Prescribed for

SUSPECTED REACTION(S) Please describe the reaction(s) and any treatment given. (Please attach additional pages if necessary):

Outcome
Recovered ☐
Recovering ☐
Continuing ☐
Other ☐

Date reaction(s) started: _____ Date reaction(s) stopped: _____
Do you consider the reactions to be serious? Yes / No
If yes, please indicate why the reaction is considered to be serious (please tick all that apply):
☐ Patient died due to reaction   ☐ Involved or prolonged inpatient hospitalisation
☐ Life threatening   ☐ Involved persistent or significant disability or incapacity
☐ Congenital abnormality   Medically significant; please give details: _____

Figure 10.6 Stopping a medication on the medication card

Regular Medications

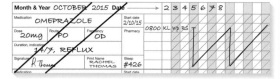

Month & Year OCTOBER 2015 Date		2	3	4	5	6	7	8	
Medication OMEPRAZOLE	Start date 2/10/15								
Dose 20mg Route PO Frequency OD Pharmacy	0800	KL	WP	RS					
Duration, indication 14/7, REFLUX									
Signature R. Thomas Print Name RACHEL THOMAS Bleep #426									
Medication	Start date								

What is a safe prescription?

A **safe prescription** is one that is **legible**, **accurate** and **relevant**. It is one where the patient has **consented** to the medications.

Before prescribing medications, **allergies** (including what the reaction was) and **contra-indications** need to have been **established**, **considered** and **documented** (Figure 10.1). If a patient develops any new allergies, these need to be added to the medication card, and treatment with suspected agents stopped. **Interactions** with other medications also need to be reviewed. Thus, the present medications need to be thoroughly reviewed prior to any additional medications being prescribed. **Comorbidities** such as **renal** and **liver failure**, and the patient's **age**, also need to be considered – these may alter how medications are metabolised, utilised and excreted, thus affecting dose frequency or size. If **calculations** to determine doses are required, ensure that you check these with a colleague.

When writing on the medication card, the writing needs to be **neat**, **legible** and in **block capital letters** in **ink**. Different information will be required by different hospitals, but the **patient name** (usually on the front and at the top of each section of the medication card), a **drug name** (usually generic), and the **route of administration**, **frequency** and **dosage** are required. A **signature**, **time** and **date** of when prescribed are also needed, and it is good

Practical Medical Procedures at a Glance, First Edition. Rachel K. Thomas © Rachel K. Thomas. Published 2015 by John Wiley & Sons, Ltd.
Companion website: http://www.ataglanceseries.com/practicalmedprocedures

practice to document in the patient's **clinical notes** which medications are started or stopped also. Medication cards are often divided into **sections**. **Regular medications** include medications prescribed upon admission, as well as medications that the patient usually takes at home (Figure 10.2). There is usually a section for medications that should be given **once only** (commonly also referred to as '**stat**' doses when the dose is to be given immediately; Figure 10.3). There are usually also sections for medications that should be given only **when required** (commonly PRN, which stands for *pro re nata*, or 'as the situation arises'; Figure 10.4).

There needs to be a clear **indication** for the medications, which is often also noted on the prescription card. An initial **duration** should also be noted. A **review date** of the medication should also be marked (Figure 10.2).

Always check **local guidelines** and **protocols**, and resources such as the **British National Formulary (BNF),** prior to prescribing medications, especially ones you are unfamiliar with. The back of the BNF also has a facility for reporting **suspected adverse drug reactions**. This is via a removable slip of paper, inside the back few pages of the book, called the **Yellow Card** (Figure 10.5).

Most Healthcare Trusts use online prescriptions, and most also have online resources to facilitate the writing of a safe prescription.

Why is a safe prescription important?

Many errors in hospital relate to prescriptions and medication. These errors can result in mild to **severe outcomes**, many of which could have been easily avoided by careful consideration when the medication chart was written up. Errors also commonly occur due to unclear handwriting, so it is advisable to write in **block capital letters** and to use only **approved abbreviations** (e.g. 'u' is not used for units, nor is 'μ' for micro).

When **stopping** a medication, it must be **fully crossed out**, dated and signed. It must be crossed out through the section for administration, as well as the section containing the prescription (Figure 10.6). Similarly, if a **new dose** for an existing medication is started, cross off the previous prescription and **rewrite** the new dose as a new and separate prescription.

Hints and tips:
- Always **check** the **BNF** and local guidelines prior to prescribing a drug you are unfamiliar with.
- Check **allergies** prior to prescribing medications, and record what the **reaction** was.
- **Ask for help** if unsure – know how to contact your senior doctors and pharmacists.
- Some hospitals will not permit doctors of certain levels to prescribe some medications (e.g. junior doctors may not be permitted to prescribe cytotoxic agents), so **check local guidelines**.
- Consider the **route** – a patient may need a cannula inserted for intravenous access (see Chapter 13).

Prescribing intravenous fluid infusions

Intravenous infusions are commonly prescribed, such as for **fluid balance maintenance** of a patient (see Chapter 16). Many hospital medication cards will have a specific section for fluid prescriptions. Assess a patient's **fluid status**, and check for signs of **cardiovascular compromise** prior to fluid prescription. It is important to specify the **time frame** (rate) over which the fluids need to be administered – for example, whilst it may be appropriate to administer a larger volume at a faster rate to a young, healthy, preoperative adult patient with electrolyte values within normal ranges and no comorbidities, a slower rate may be appropriate for an elderly patient with heart failure and hypernatraemia. Resources such as the **National Institute for Clinical Excellence (NICE)** have guidelines available for the prescription of fluids.

Prescribing blood and blood product infusions

Blood and **blood product infusions** are another type of fluid infusion, although less frequently prescribed (see Chapter 17). According to each hospital's policies, they may be prescribed within an infusion section, or a specific **transfusion section** of the medication card. Again, a **duration** needs to be indicated – for example, 4-hourly for red blood cells – however, this must be based on the clinical indication and an assessment of the patient's **fluid status** and **cardiovascular system**.

Prescribing oxygen

Oxygen is a **medication** and therefore must be **prescribed**. Most hospitals will have a dedicated section on the medication card for this (see Chapter 21). Be sure to first confirm the patient's clinical requirements and comorbidities. Normally, target oxygen saturations are **94–98%**. However, in conditions such as **chronic obstructive pulmonary disease (COPD)**, patients may have a lower target oxygen saturation level of **88–92%**, and these desired **target saturations** should be recorded. The delivery device needs to be specified, be it a **nasal cannula**, **Venturi mask**, **simple face mask** (also referred to as a Hudson mask) or **non-rebreather mask** (see Chapter 21). The flow **rate** may need to be indicated, as well as whether the oxygen is to be given **intermittently** (or PRN, i.e. 'as required') or **continuously**. **Nebulisers** and **inhalers** must also be prescribed (see Chapter 22).

Prescribing syringe drivers and patient-controlled analgesia

Syringe drivers are small pumps used to administer medications gradually. They are commonly used for pain relief, such as for morphine delivery in a palliative care setting. When prescribing, ensure that the **additives**, the **dose** and the **diluent** are specified, and ensure the **compatibility** of the components. The medication can be delivered **subcutaneously** or **intravenously** via the driver, over a specified timeframe.

Patient-controlled analgesia (PCA) consists of **bolus doses** of medication being administered **intravenously**, via a button pressed by the patient, with a system that will '**lock out**', preventing an overdose. Ensure that the patient is not on any other opioid pain medications, as it may accumulate if given concurrently, and it is good practice to also prescribe naloxone in the PRN section of the card in case of opioid overdose.

Both delivery systems are a specific type of prescription, which usually has a **dedicated region** of the medication card. They should be prescribed with more **specialised knowledge**, and **reviewed frequently**.

Did you know?
Common abbreviations:
- Timing –
  OD – once per day (24-hourly)
  BD – twice per day (12-hourly)
  TDS – three times per day (8-hourly)
  QDS – four times per day (6-hourly)
  PRN – as required
  OM – every morning
  ON – every night
- Duration –
  /7 – days
  /52 – weeks
  ° – hourly
- Route –
  PO – orally
  PR – rectally
  IV – intravenously
  IM – intramuscularly
  SC – subcutaneously

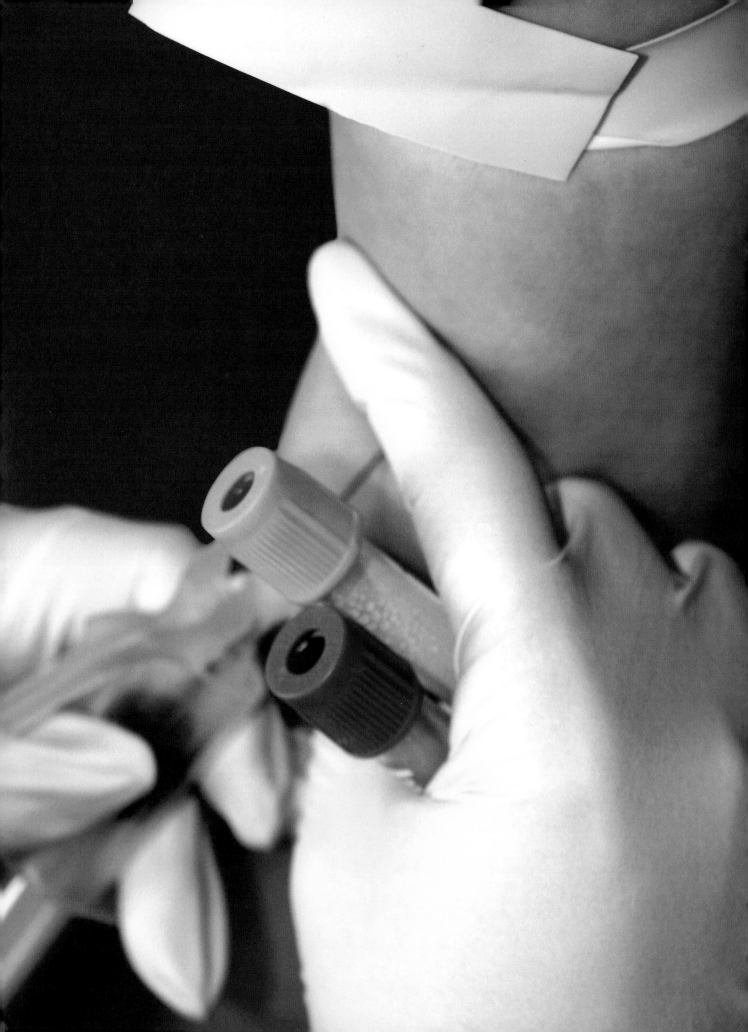

Common invasive ward procedures

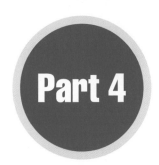

Part 4

Chapters

11 Performing venepuncture 28
12 Taking blood cultures 30
13 Inserting a cannula in a peripheral vein 32
14 Measuring blood glucose 34
15 Suturing 36

11 Performing venepuncture

Figure 11.1 Examples of different equipment for taking blood: a butterfly needle, a safety needle and a cannula and Vacutainer® adapters

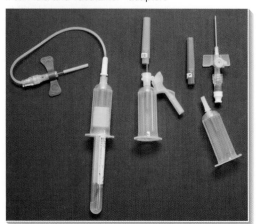

Figure 11.2 A typical request form

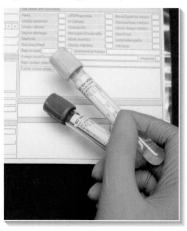

Figure 11.3 A sample of draw order

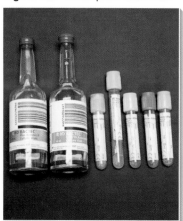

Figure 11.4 Veins of the ante-cubital fossa. Source: Stephenson et al (2013).

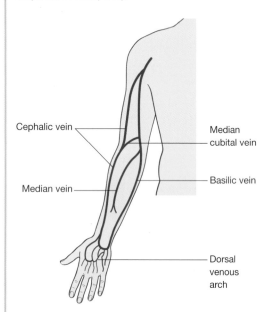

Cephalic vein

Median cubital vein

Basilic vein

Median vein

Dorsal venous arch

Did you know?

Blood sample bottle colours differ according to local policies, so ensure you become familiar with them. For example:
- Red – serum samples, thyroid, B_{12}
- Pink – cross-match, G&S
- Blue – international normalisation ratio (INR), clotting
- Yellow/green – biochemistry, urea and electrolytes, liver function tests
- Purple – full blood count
- Grey – glucose

Hints and tips:

- Always adhere to **local protocols** where available.
- Select veins by gentle **palpation**, not by vision.
- **Needle stick** injuries need to be **washed, bleeding encouraged**, and **Occupational Health notified** for local policies for further actions (see Chapter 3).
- Only use syringes if unavoidable – they are more dangerous, expensive and have greater lab rejection rates.
- Ensure you have immediate access to a **sharps disposal container**, prior to starting.

Figure 11.5 Equipment for venepuncture

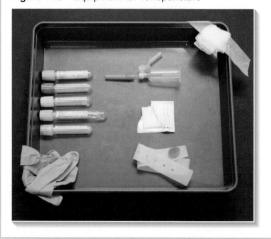

Figure 11.6 Taking a blood sample

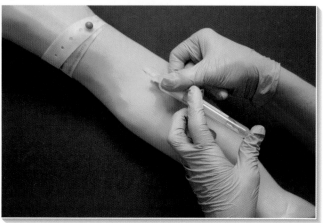

Practical Medical Procedures at a Glance, First Edition. Rachel K. Thomas © Rachel K. Thomas. Published 2015 by John Wiley & Sons, Ltd.
Companion website: http://www.ataglanceseries.com/practicalmedprocedures

What is venepuncture?

Venepuncture, or taking blood, is a skill that is best mastered early on. It is a daily occurrence in a hospital setting. It can be taken with special collection systems such as the **Vacutainer® needle** (or **Vacutainer butterfly needle** for smaller veins or **Vacutainer** adaptors from a cannula; Figure 11.1). The blood is collected in colour-coded vials and sent to Biochemistry, Haematology or Microbiology for processing, along with the appropriate investigation requests. These **request forms** may be on paper or via an online system, depending on local protocols (Figure 11.2). All vials have a **vacuum**, which facilitates the collection of a predetermined volume of blood. Some vials have **additives**, such as anticoagulants or gels, which are required for the specific testing of some samples.

Blood can also be taken with a **needle and syringe**; however, this method should be used as a **last resort**, due to greater laboratory rejection rates of the acquired samples, lower safety levels (a greater risk of **needle-stick injuries**) and greater cost.

Why is venepuncture important?

Blood samples are required for **diagnosis** of conditions, for **monitoring** of therapy and for **measurement** of medication levels (e.g. gentamicin and phenytoin).

Always take care with the **order of draw** for blood samples. The **additives** of some tubes can alter the results of other tubes filled later by **contamination**. Therefore, always draw in the specified order, as per local Healthcare Trust protocols as colours and draw orders may vary (Figure 11.3). Also, some bottles, such as the coagulation sample (often a blue bottle), need to be **filled** to the **specified marker**.

If you are **unsuccessful** in collecting the blood, explain to the patient, and **retry** with a new set of equipment if they are happy for you to do so. If not, either return later, or request your supervisor to try, depending on the urgency of the situation.

Indications
- Measurement of physiological parameters and diagnosis
- Monitoring drug levels and therapy effects

Contra-indications
- Patient refusal
- Arteriovenous fistula
- Infection at site

Complications
- **Local** – pain and/or bruising at site, infection, haematoma
- **Systemic** – fainting

Aspects of vein selection

Selecting a good vein is vital. Veins should be selected by how they **feel** (**gentle palpation**). If they are palpated too firmly, most veins will collapse. Selecting by visual appearance can be deceptive, as the visible veins may not necessarily be of suitable size or volume. Through palpation with **two fingers** or the thumb, it should feel springy when the pressure put on it with the fingers is **released**. Any veins can be used, although those most commonly used are in the antecubital fossa of the **non-dominant hand** (Figure 11.4).

Various measures can be taken to help with finding a vein after applying a **tourniquet** to encourage venous engorgement. Simple measures using **gravity** (e.g. hanging the patient's arm down) can help, as can **warming** the hand in water. Repeatedly **making a fist**, by clenching and reopening the hand, can also help. Always remember to check for patient comfort, as, for instance, a patient with arthritis of the hand may find repeatedly making a fist painful. Ensure that the region to be sampled is **well supported**, such as by resting the arm on a pillow.

Avoid taking blood from veins that are part of an **arteriovenous fistula** (A-V fistula, a surgically created join between an artery and a vein, for the purpose of dialysis), and those which have a **cannula** already near them (see Chapter 13). Avoid taking blood from an arm that has **intravenous fluids** running into it (commonly referred to as a 'drip arm'), as this will influence the values obtained (see Chapter 16).

Try to avoid **valves** in the vein, which may feel **firmer** and slightly knobbly. A **thrombosis** in the **vein** will be **hard**, and these should also be avoided. Also avoid **arteries**, which will be **pulsatile**. Look carefully to ensure that there is no venous inflammation (phlebitis), which may be visible as a **redness** following the path of the vein. Also look for any **bruising**, **wounds** or **skin infection**, and avoid these sites if possible.

Did you know?
- Once a **Vacutainer®** vial seal has been broken, it will no longer collect the blood if it has lost its **negative pressure**. This may be a reason for failure; use a new vial.

Procedure

- **Introduce** yourself, and **identify** the patient (see Chapter 4).
- Gain **consent** for the procedure (see Chapter 5), explain **indications** and check for **contra-indications** or **allergies**.
- Ensure **bare below the elbows**, and **wash hands** (see Chapter 6).
- Wipe clean a **tray** with antibacterial wipes. Collect equipment (Figure 11.5), and place in tray using the **aseptic non-touch technique (ANTT)** (see Chapter 8), including:
  - Non-sterile gloves
  - Vacutainer® collection system
  - Needle or butterfly needle
  - Tourniquet (preferably single use)
  - Chlorhexidine wipe
  - Blood sample vials
  - Dressing and swab.
- **Assemble the Vacutainer® collection** system and **needle or butterfly needle** using **ANTT**, hence without touching **key parts**.
- Ensure that the patient is **comfortable**, with the area to have blood taken from well supported with a pillow.
- Apply a **tourniquet**, and palpate the vein distal to the tourniquet – select the vein by **palpation**, not by visual appearance.
- **Wash hands**, and put on **gloves**. Tighten the tourniquet if it has been loosened.
- **Anchor vein, clean** with chlorhexidine wipe and allow to **air dry**.
- **Avoid re-palpation** at the intended site of puncture, as this is a **key site**, and **anchor or tether vein** below this site.
- Warn patient of a **sharp scratch**; confidently insert the needle, which is held in your dominant hand at a **less than 45° angle** with the **bevel up**; and minimise needle movement (Figure 11.6).
- **Attach sample bottles** in the correct order according to local protocols (Figure 11.3) using your non-dominant hand to attach the bottles, with your dominant hand stabilising the needle.
- **Release tourniquet, withdraw needle**, apply swab with pressure for a minute (or longer, if still bleeding) and apply dressing over the puncture site.
- **Safely dispose of sharps** (after activating a **needle safety device**, if present) in a clinical sharps bins.
- Dispose of waste in a clinical waste bin, and clean the tray.
- Remove gloves, and **wash hands**.
- Label specimens with the patient's name, hospital number, date of birth and all relevant required information, including a bleep number. **Do not leave unlabelled samples unattended**.
- **Document** in the patient's notes date, time, signature, designation and any difficulties encountered.
- **Thank patient**, and ensure that they are comfortable and have no adverse effects.
- Ensure samples are sent to the correct departments.

12 Taking blood cultures

Figure 12.1 Signs of sepsis

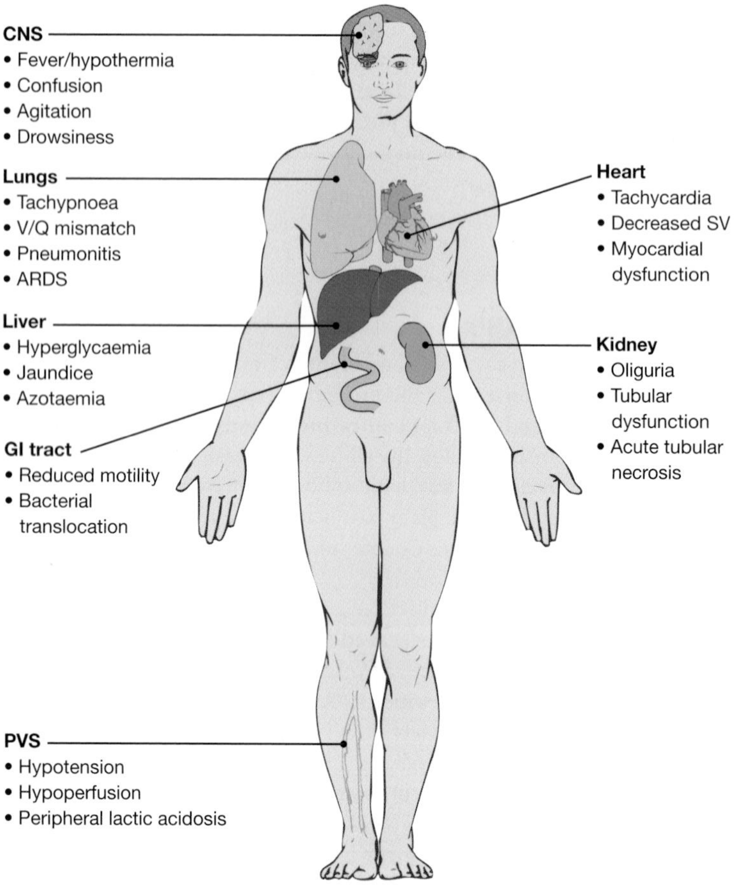

CNS
- Fever/hypothermia
- Confusion
- Agitation
- Drowsiness

Lungs
- Tachypnoea
- V/Q mismatch
- Pneumonitis
- ARDS

Liver
- Hyperglycaemia
- Jaundice
- Azotaemia

GI tract
- Reduced motility
- Bacterial translocation

PVS
- Hypotension
- Hypoperfusion
- Peripheral lactic acidosis

Heart
- Tachycardia
- Decreased SV
- Myocardial dysfunction

Kidney
- Oliguria
- Tubular dysfunction
- Acute tubular necrosis

Figure 12.2 Equipment for taking blood cultures

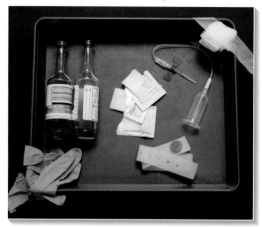

Hints and tips:
- Take the **aerobic** sample prior to the **anaerobic** sample.
- Wipe the top of the bottle with a **chlorhexidine wipe** prior to collecting sample.
- Collect as large a blood sample as possible – the bottles are a vacuum. Aim for **8 to 10 ml**.
- Remember that signs of **sepsis** may be decreased in the paediatric and the elderly patient.
- If further blood samples are required, take them **after** the blood culture samples have been collected.

Figure 12.3 Clean the top of the bottle prior to sample collection

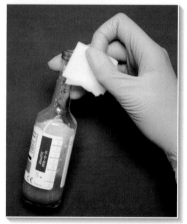

Figure 12.4 Aerobic and anaerobic blood culture bottles

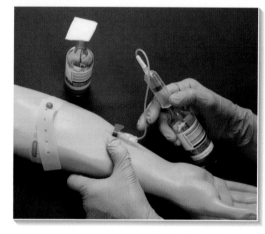

Practical Medical Procedures at a Glance, First Edition. Rachel K. Thomas © Rachel K. Thomas. Published 2015 by John Wiley & Sons, Ltd.
Companion website: http://www.ataglanceseries.com/practicalmedprocedures

What are blood cultures?

Blood cultures are samples of **blood** that are sent to **Microbiology**, where they are processed to help determine the presence of **infection**. There are two types of blood cultures – **aerobic** and **anaerobic**. **Aerobic** samples must be taken **first** (to test for organisms which live with exposure to **oxygen**), followed by **anaerobic** samples (for organisms which live only **without oxygen** exposure). Some hospital protocols require only aerobic samples, unless certain conditions such as endocarditis are suspected, and then these protocols will also stipulate the number of cultures required for diagnosis – for example, three sets of positive cultures.

The bottles required for taking the blood cultures have **expiry dates**, which need to be checked prior to use.

Many hospitals will have **blood culture packs** which contain all the required equipment, as there are strict regulations on the usage of **Vacutainer**® collection systems and **butterfly needles**. This is to minimise the risk of contamination, and maximise the chances of successful sample collection.

Why are blood cultures important?

Blood cultures are required in cases where the patient may have an **infection**. They can help isolate the **cause** of the infection, and then test how **sensitive** the organism is to various antibiotics. Therefore, they should be considered in a patient with a **raised temperature**, and they are best taken during a **temperature spike**. However, they should only be taken if there is **clinical indication** or suspicion of blood infection (septicaemia). They are often part of a '**septic screen**' (see Chapter 9). There are **many signs** of sepsis (Figure 12.1). These signs may present differently in various patients, such as in paediatric and elderly patients.

The collection bottles are **vacuumed**, and you should aim to collect as much blood as possible, as this increases the chances of culturing the organism. You should aim to collect preferably **8–10 ml of blood** in each collection bottle.

Many hospitals will have **protocols** in place, such as empirical antibiotic treatment, which should be commenced immediately after the cultures have been taken. Once a patient is already on **antibiotics**, the taking of blood cultures is less useful.

Indications
- Elevated temperature
- Clinical suspicion of infection or sepsis

Contra-indications
- Patient refusal
- Arteriovenous fistula
- Infection at site

Complications
- **Local** – pain, bruising, infection
- **Systemic** – infection

Procedure
- **Introduce** yourself, and **identify** the patient (see Chapter 4).
- Gain **consent** for the procedure (see Chapter 5), explain **indications** and check for **contra-indications**.
- Ensure **bare below the elbows**, and **wash hands** (see Chapter 6).
- Wipe clean a **tray** with antibacterial wipes.

- Collect equipment (Figure 12.2), and place in tray using the **aseptic non-touch technique (ANTT)** (see Chapter 8), including:
  - Non-sterile gloves
  - Vacutainer® collection system
  - Butterfly needle
  - Tourniquet (preferably single use)
  - Chlorhexidine wipes
  - Blood culture bottles
  - Dressing and swab.
- **Clean top** of blood culture bottles with **chlorhexidine**; wipe after removal of plastic cap (Figure 12.3).
- Assemble **Vacutainer collection system** and **butterfly needle**, using **ANTT** and thus not touching **key parts**.
- Ensure that the patient is **comfortable**, with the area to have blood taken from well supported with a pillow.
- Apply the **tourniquet**, palpate the vein distal to the tourniquet – select a vein by **palpation**, not by visual appearance. Once a suitable vein has been **identified**, the tourniquet can be loosened.
- **Anchor or tether vein**, **clean** with a chlorhexidine wipe and allow to **air dry**.
- **Wash hands**, and put on **gloves**. Tighten the tourniquet if it has been loosened.
- **Avoid re-palpation** at the intended site of puncture, as this is a **key site**, and **anchor vein** below this site.
- Warn the patient of a **sharp scratch**, confidently insert the needle at a **less than 45° angle** with the **bevel up** and minimise needle movement.
- Fill blood culture bottles – **aerobic first, anaerobic second** – by attaching the bottles individually to the **Vacutainer collection** set (Figure 12.4). Collect as much blood as possible in the vacuumed bottle, preferably 8–10 ml.
- Keep bottle **upright** whilst collecting the sample.
- **Agitate** bottles once filled with the sample.
- **Release tourniquet**, **withdraw needle**, apply swab with pressure for a minute (or longer, if still bleeding) and apply **dressing** over the puncture site.
- **Safely dispose of sharps** (after activating the **needle safety device**, if present) in clinical sharps bins.
- Dispose of waste in clinical waste bins, and clean tray.
- Remove gloves and **wash hands**.
- **Label** specimens with the patient's name, hospital number, date of birth and all relevant required information, including a bleep number. **Do not leave unlabelled samples unattended**.
- **Document** in the patient's notes date, time, signature, designation and any difficulties encountered. Place sticker in the notes, from blood culture bottles, if present.
- **Thank patient**, and ensure that they are comfortable and have no adverse effects.
- Ensure samples are sent to the **Microbiology** department.
- Continue with **hospital protocol** for management, such as starting empirical antibiotics if this is indicated.

Did you know?
Severe sepsis requires the **Sepsis Six** to be started immediately, and definitely within **1 hour**:
1. High-flow oxygen
2. Intravenous fluids
3. Blood samples, including cultures
4. Lactate levels
5. Antibiotics
6. Hourly urine monitoring

13 Inserting a cannula in a peripheral vein

Figure 13.1 Angle of cannula insertion

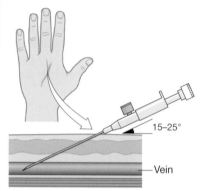

15–25°

Vein

Figure 13.3 Equipment required for cannula insertion

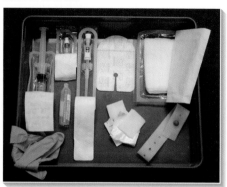

Figure 13.4 Intravenous cannula sizes

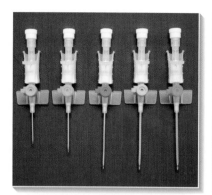

Figure 13.2
Key parts, circled, must not be touched

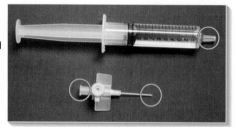

Figure 13.5
Cannula insertion

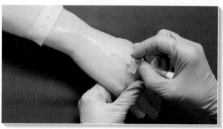

Hints and Tips:

- **Never touch key parts.**
- An **ultrasound probe** can be useful to help cannulate difficult veins.
- Remember to always **flush** the cannula, and needle-free bung with **saline prior** to use, and to check for 'tissuing' (fluid seepage into the surrounding tissue).
- **Blood samples** can be taken only when the cannula is **first inserted** – use a Vacutainer ® connector system and ANTT.
- The **larger** the bore, the **smaller** the gauge number and the **faster** the delivery of the fluids.
- When removing the needle, consider applying **pressure** to the vein immediately **proximal** to the cannula to decrease the blood flow.

Figure 13.6 Visual Infusion Phlebitis score. Source: Dr K Nagaratnam and Dr E Torok, IV access working group, Oxford University Hospitals NHS Trust. Reproduced with permission of Dr K Nagaratnam.

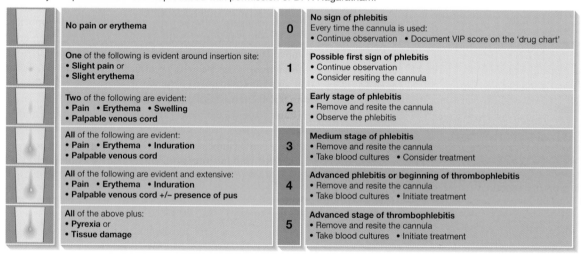

	No pain or erythema	0	**No sign of phlebitis** Every time the cannula is used: • Continue observation • Document VIP score on the 'drug chart'
	One of the following is evident around insertion site: • **Slight pain** or • **Slight erythema**	1	**Possible first sign of phlebitis** • Continue observation • Consider resiting the cannula
	Two of the following are evident: • **Pain** • **Erythema** • **Swelling** • **Palpable venous cord**	2	**Early stage of phlebitis** • Remove and resite the cannula • Observe the phlebitis
	All of the following are evident: • **Pain** • **Erythema** • **Induration** • **Palpable venous cord**	3	**Medium stage of phlebitis** • Remove and resite the cannula • Take blood cultures • Consider treatment
	All of the following are evident and extensive: • **Pain** • **Erythema** • **Induration** • **Palpable venous cord** +/– **presence of pus**	4	**Advanced phlebitis or beginning of thrombophlebitis** • Remove and resite the cannula • Take blood cultures • Initiate treatment
	All of the above plus: • **Pyrexia** or • **Tissue damage**	5	**Advanced stage of thrombophlebitis** • Remove and resite the cannula • Take blood cultures • Initiate treatment

What is a cannula?

A **cannula** is a needle with a **fine plastic tube** around it, which is inserted into the patient's **vein** (Figure 13.1). The needle is then removed, and the plastic tube remains in the vessel, **secured** into place externally with a **sterile dressing**. It is a **mini surgical procedure**, and thus needs meticulous attention to asepsis (see Chapter 8). **Key parts must not be touched** – these include the **tip** of the **flush**, the **syringe** and the **bung** (Figure 13.2). It is recommended that the packages be

Practical Medical Procedures at a Glance, First Edition. Rachel K. Thomas © Rachel K. Thomas. Published 2015 by John Wiley & Sons, Ltd.
Companion website: http://www.ataglanceseries.com/practicalmedprocedures

opened in preparation, but that the key parts remain inside the inner sterile surfaces of their packages until used (Figure 13.3).

Why is cannulation important?

Cannulation is performed to give **access** to the circulatory system, for the delivery of **fluid**, **medications** and **blood**. **Different sizes** of cannulae are available, depending on the clinical scenario, such as the required speed of delivery and the patient's anatomy (Figure 13.4).

The cannula can be left *in situ* for several days, provided there are no signs of infection, enabling intravenous delivery over **longer durations**, and sparing the patient **repeated injections**. It is therefore important to consider choosing a **site** which will cause **minimal discomfort** for the patient, such as the back of the hand, if this is clinically appropriate (Figure 13.5). Many local protocols contra-indicate their insertion in the same side as previous breast surgery.

Blood samples can be collected when a cannula is first inserted. If **blood samples** are required, attach a **Vacutainer®** connector (adaptor) using the **aseptic non-touch technique (ANTT) prior to flushing the cannula** (see Chapter 11).

Infection signs around cannulae are monitored and recorded as part of protocols in most hospitals. Ensure that you document any signs of infection, and adhere to local policies such as Visual Infusion Phlebitis (VIP) scores, if they are in place (Figure 13.6). A cannula needs to be **removed** and **replaced** if signs of phlebitis or infection are present.

Indications
- Administration of intravenous fluids, blood, medications

Contra-indications
- Patient refusal
- Arteriovenous fistula
- Infection at site

Complications
- **Local** – 'tissuing', phlebitis, infection, pain
- **Systemic** – infection, air embolism

Procedure

- **Introduce** yourself, and **identify** the patient (see Chapter 4).
- Gain **consent** for the procedure (see Chapter 5), explain **indications** and check for **contra-indications** or **allergies**.
- Ensure **bare below the elbows**, and **wash hands** (see Chapter 6).
- Wipe clean a **tray** with antibacterial wipes.
- Collect equipment (Figure 13.3) and place in tray using the **aseptic non-touch technique (ANTT)** (see Chapter 8), including:
  - Non-sterile gloves
  - Cannula
  - Needle-free bung/extension set
  - Tourniquet (preferably single use)
  - Chlorhexidine wipes
  - For saline flush: saline solution for injection
    Drawing up needle
    10 ml syringe
  - Sterile cannula dressing
  - Swabs.

Preparing the saline flush:
- Connect the **drawing-up needle** to the **syringe** using ANTT, not touching the tip of the syringe or the base of the needle as these are **key parts** (see Chapter 8).
- Check **saline name**, **expiry date**, and **lot number**, and open the vial.

- **Insert needle** into the saline solution, and draw up into the syringe by pulling back on the syringe plunger.
- **Expel** any air left in the syringe by slowly pressing the plunger into the syringe, whilst simultaneously **tapping the side** of the syringe.
- **Safely dispose of sharps** in clinical sharps bins.
- **Flush needle-free bung/extension set** (as detailed below).
- Place saline-filled syringe inside tray, with the tip of the syringe replaced inside the **original sterile packaging**.

Preparing the needle-free bung/extension set:
- **Open bung/extension set** package using ANTT, taking care not to touch the ends as these are **key parts**.
- **Flush** with saline by attaching the syringe to each terminal port and slowly depressing the plunger, taking care to not touch the **key parts**.
- Replace inside the **original sterile packaging** (Figure 13.3).

Inserting the cannula:
- Ensure that the patient is **comfortable**, with the area to be cannulated well supported by a pillow, resting on a linen saver.
- Apply **tourniquet**, and palpate the vein distal to the tourniquet – select a vein by **palpation**, not by visual appearance.
- **Slightly loosen the tourniquet**.
- **Wash hands**, and put on **gloves**.
- **Unsheathe** the cannula, fold **open** the side grips and ensure that all the equipment is ready to use.
- **Tighten the tourniquet**.
- **Anchor or tether vein with non-dominant hand**, clean with a chlorhexidine wipe and allow to **air dry for 30 seconds**.
- Pick up the cannula with preferred grip in your dominant hand, and slide the needle back and then forward slightly within the plastic cannula tube to ensure it is moving freely. **Do not touch key parts!**
- **Avoid re-palpation** at the intended site of puncture, as this is a **key site**; **anchor vein** below this site.
- Warn patient of a '**sharp scratch**', and confidently insert needle at a **15–25° degree angle** with the bevel up, minimising needle movement (Figure 13.1).
- Observe for **primary flashback** in the **window** at the back of the cannula.
- **Flatten** the angle of insertion, and **advance** the cannula a few millimetres beyond the point of flashback (Figure 13.5).
- Retract the needle whilst observing for **secondary flashback** in the **lumen** of the cannula; slide the cannula over the needle into the vein, whilst maintaining the traction to the skin.
- **Release** the tourniquet, whilst occluding the proximal end of the cannula on the skin.
- **Remove needle**, and **safely dispose** of it in a clinical sharps bin.
- **Attach needle-free bung, without touching key parts**.
- **Flush cannula** with the **saline**, to ensure it is sited accurately and to decrease clot formation, by attaching the saline-filled syringe to the bung/extension set and slowly depressing the plunger.
- Secure cannula with **sterile dressing**.
- Dispose of waste in clinical waste bins, **safely dispose of sharps** in clinical sharps bins, and clean tray.
- Remove gloves, and **wash hands**.
- **Record** in the notes and patient medication card the cannula insertion time, date, signature, name and designation, and any difficulties encountered.
- **Record VIP score** in the patient's medication card, or according to local protocol (Figure 13.6).
- **Thank patient**, and ensure that they are comfortable and have no adverse effects.

14 Measuring blood glucose

Figure 14.1 The test strip and handheld glucose monitor

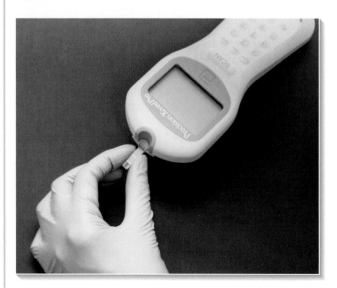

Figure 14.2 Pricking the finger to obtain a drop of blood for testing

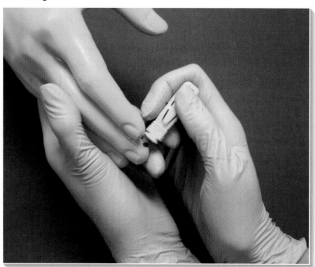

Figure 14.3 Dispose of your lancet in the sharps bin

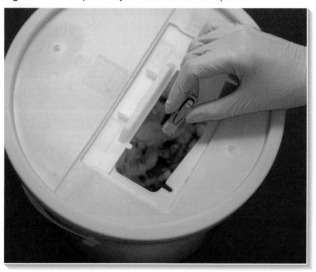

Figure 14.4 Collection of sample onto test strip

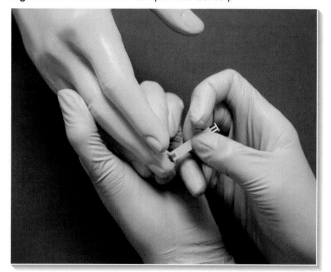

Hints and tips:

- Capillary glucose measurements can be inaccurate and need to be confirmed by a **plasma glucose** sample in the **laboratory**.
- Make sure the patient's hand is socially **clean** as alcohol swabbing on the fingertip may alter the results.
- **Warm hands** will help the blood flow.
- Prick the **side** of the fingertip on any of the third, fourth and fifth fingers of the non-dominant hand rather than the pulp as the latter is more sensitive.

Did you know?

- **Hyperglycaemia** may present with polyuria, polydipsia, confusion and coma.

  In diabetic **ketoacidosis (DKA)**, the patient may also exhibit Kussmaul (sighing) respiration, abdominal pain, nausea, vomiting and diarrhoea.
- **Hypoglycaemia** may present with sweating, pallor, tachycardia, palpitations, tremor (autonomic origins), irritability, anger, confusion, coma (neurological origins).

Practical Medical Procedures at a Glance, First Edition. Rachel K. Thomas © Rachel K. Thomas. Published 2015 by John Wiley & Sons, Ltd.
Companion website: http://www.ataglanceseries.com/practicalmedprocedures

What is blood glucose measurement?

A 'blood glucose' measurement – or, more accurately, a 'capillary glucose' measurement – is a simple test used to determine the approximate level of **glucose** in a person's **blood**. It is a quick test and, while not as accurate as measuring the plasma glucose level in a laboratory sample, it is extremely useful, particularly in **emergency** situations as the result is obtained on the spot. Normal fasting blood glucose levels are between 4 and 6 mmol/L. Above this level, it is **hyperglycaemia**; below this level, it is **hypoglycaemia**.

Did you know?

Blood glucose is frequently referred to as a **BM** – this is because the company that invented the kit was called Boehringer Mannheim.

Why are blood glucose measurements important?

A blood glucose level is used both in **acute settings** in hospital and in the management of **chronic diseases** in the community. Blood glucose levels need to be maintained as close to the physiological norm as possible, in order to minimise the development of other complications. A suspected diagnosis of diabetes should be confirmed with a **plasma glucose level test**. If a random glucose level is ≥11.0 mmol/l, or a fasting glucose level is ≥7.0 mmol/L, this is sufficient for a diagnosis of diabetes. If a random plasma glucose level is elevated but does not reach the criteria for diabetes, an **oral glucose tolerance test** can be carried out.

Indications
- Investigation of any unconscious patient, seizures, sepsis
- Diabetes investigation and management, pancreatitis

Contra-indications
- Patient refusal

Complications
- **Local** – pain and/or bruising at site
- **Systemic** – fainting

Procedure

- **Introduce** yourself, and **identify** the patient (see Chapter 4).
- Gain **consent** for the procedure (see Chapter 5), explain **indications** and check for **contra-indications** or **allergies**.
- Ensure **bare below the elbows**, and **wash hands** (see Chapter 6).
- Ensure that the **patient has clean hands**.
- Wipe clean a **tray** with antibacterial wipes.
- Collect equipment and place it in a tray, including:
  - Non-sterile gloves
  - Spring-loaded lancing device
  - Handheld glucose monitor (calibrated)
  - Swab
  - Test strip.
- Check **expiry date** on strips.
- Prepare the strip and device for specimen collection by removing the outer packaging and inserting the strip into the handheld device.
- **Wash hands**, and put on **gloves**.
- Follow the instructions on the handheld device, scanning the patient's identification (ID) bracelet and your own ID if required.
- **Avoid touching the reagent part of the strip whilst inserting into device** (Figure 14.1).
- **Warn the patient that there will be a sharp sting.**
- Lance the **side** of the pulp space of the ring or little finger of the patient's non-dominant hand (Figure 14.2).
- **Safely dispose of the lancet** in the **clinical sharps bin** (Figure 14.3).
- Obtain a specimen by holding the end of the test strip against the drop of blood and allowing the blood to **soak** into the strip – ensure that it soaks in fully (Figure 14.4).
- Stem the blood flow with a swab.
- Thank the patient, and ensure that they are comfortable and have no adverse effects.
- Remove gloves, and **wash hands**.
- **Document** the result in the **patient notes**, including result, date, time, designation, signature, contact details and any **problems** that may have been encountered.
- If appropriate, manage hyper- and hypoglycaemia according to local Healthcare Trust protocols.

15 Suturing

Figure 15.1 Types of sutures

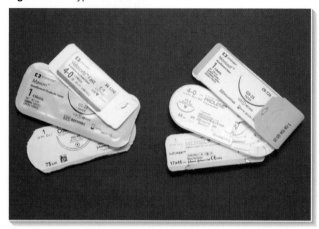

Figure 15.2 Types of needles

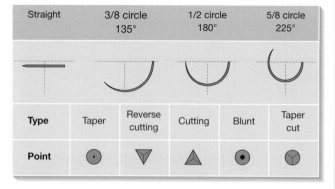

	Straight	3/8 circle 135°	1/2 circle 180°	5/8 circle 225°	
Type	Taper	Reverse cutting	Cutting	Blunt	Taper cut
Point	⊙	▽	△	⦿	⅄

Figure 15.3 Steps in an interrupted suture

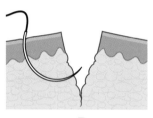

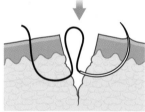

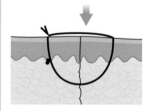

Box 15.1 Common suture types

- Absorbable:
  - Vicryl
  - Monocryl
- Non-absorbable:
  - Silk
  - Prolene

Figure 15.4 Suturing equipment

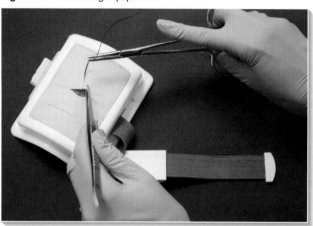

Did you know?

Non-absorbable sutures are removed at different times, depending on factors such as location, wound type, depth, and comorbidities such as diabetes. Always advise patients of an estimated time for removal:

Face	4–7 days
Scalp	7–10 days
Limbs	10–14 days

Figure 15.5 Protecting the needle

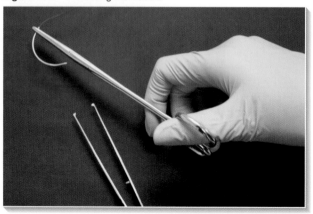

Hints and tips:
- Always use **ANTT**.
- Establish the **time** and **mechanism** of injury
- Establish whether the patient is anti-coagulated.
- When not in use, twist the needle so that the sharp end is **protected** by the forceps.
- Remember to check **tetanus** status.
- Remember to **remove non-viable tissue**.
- Inform the patient of signs of **inflammation**, and ensure that they understand when to **seek further medical help**.
- Consider closure methods such as **steri-strips**, **glue** and **staples**.
- Check for any **neurovascular deficit** prior to suturing.

Practical Medical Procedures at a Glance, First Edition. Rachel K. Thomas © Rachel K. Thomas. Published 2015 by John Wiley & Sons, Ltd.
Companion website: http://www.ataglanceseries.com/practicalmedprocedures

What are sutures?

Suturing and basic knot tying are skills that have many applications and need to be **practised frequently** to become proficient. Suture material is packaged in **sterile packets**, where the suture material is swaged onto the base of an eyeless needle, thus presenting a single piece (Figure 15.1). Information regarding the type of material and needle is printed on the packet. **Instruments** used for suturing include needle holders, tissue forceps (toothed) and scissors.

There are **different classifications** of sutures – **absorbable** sutures (e.g. vicryl, polydioxanone (PDS) and monocryl) do not need removal (Box 15.1). **Non-absorbable** sutures (e.g. silk and Prolene) do require removal after the wound has healed adequately. Sutures may also be classified as **synthetic** (monocryl, vicryl, PDS or Prolene) or **non-synthetic** (silk).

Sutures are also classified into **monofilament** which consists of a single smooth strand (nylon, Prolene or monocryl) which slides through tissues with less friction and is associated with less infection, or **multifilament** (silk or vicryl) which is easier to tie and produces knots that are less likely to slip.

There are also **different grades** of coarseness of suture, for different areas. **Fine sutures** are used for areas such as the face, while **course sutures** are appropriate for securing drains and lines.

The types of **needles** used to suture vary, with **cutting needles** being used for skin, and **taper or smooth needles** for soft tissue such as the bowel or blood vessels. Needles can be semi-circular or straight (Figure 15.2).

There are **different techniques** for suturing – the most common is the **interrupted suture** (Figure 15.3). Also commonly used are sub-cuticular sutures (for optimal cosmetic results), continuous sutures (for longer wounds) and vertical sutures (for deeper wounds), which are beyond the scope of this book.

Why is suturing important?

Suturing is used to keep the edges of a **wound together** and **tension free** so that it can heal. Suturing is used when other forms of wound closure, such as **staples**, **glue** and **steri-strips**, are not clinically appropriate. Suturing is used to close skin wounds or incisions, and also to close deeper layers of anatomy. It is also used to keep lines and drains securely in the correct location.

Where you suture has a big impact on the final cosmetic result for the patient. When closing **elective incisions** from surgery, it is preferable to have the closure lines along the **natural folds** and creases of the body and face, as this minimises the appearance of scars. **Accidental wounds** are obviously less likely to fall only on these lines, and thus tend to have a worse cosmetic outcome.

Different types of wound require different closure methods. Some wounds should *not* be closed immediately with sutures, such as those at great risk of infection like animal bites. These may require cleaning, antibiotics and closure at a later time.

Suturing should be performed after **local anaesthetic** has been infiltrated (see Chapter 19).

Indications
- Wound, muscle and tissue closure
- Fixation of medical equipment –drains, lines, devices

Contra-indications
- Patient refusal
- Dirty wound – bite, infection, necrosis

Complications
- **Local** – scarring, wound dehiscence, infection
- **Systemic** – infection

Procedure

- **Introduce** yourself, and **identify** the patient (see Chapter 4).
- Gain **consent** for the procedure (see Chapter 5), explain **indications** and check for **contra-indications** or **allergies**.
- Check **tetanus status**, and consider a tetanus booster and antibiotics if appropriate.
- Ensure **bare below the elbows**, and **wash hands** (see Chapter 6).
- Wipe clean a **tray** with antibacterial wipes.
- Collect equipment and place in a tray using the **aseptic non-touch technique (ANTT)** (see Chapter 8), including:
  - A wound pack, if available
  - Toothed forceps
  - Needle holder
  - Scissors
  - Appropriate suture material
  - Irrigation fluid
  - Sterile dressing
  - Local anaesthetic syringe (see Chapter 19)
  - Sterile gloves.
- Place a **protective sheet** under the wound.
- Don apron, **wash hands** and put on **sterile gloves**.
- **Assess** wound, and select the most appropriate equipment.
- Administer **local anaesthetic** with an **intradermal injection** after checking **allergies** and after reviewing local procedure protocols (see Chapter 19). Ensure enough time passes for this to be effective – usually approximately 10 minutes.
- Thoroughly **irrigate wound**, and **remove non-viable tissue**.
- **Remove** any **foreign bodies** in the wound, look for signs of infection and clean the wound.
- Open the suture package, and, holding the **needle** two-thirds from the tip, mount in **needle holder**.
- Using **toothed forceps**, **lift** the skin on one side of the wound, in the centre of the wound (Figure 15.4). Do not crush tissue.
- Insert the needle at a **90° angle**, through the skin, and out into the **middle** of the wound (Figure 15.3).
- **Release** the needle holder hold on the needle, and **re-grasp** the needle in the centre of the wound.
- **Re-pierce** the wound from the **inside**, and pass it through the skin out onto the skin on the other side.
- Re-secure the needle with the needle holder, ensuring that the pointed section is **protected** (Figure 15.5).
- **Knot** the thread by hand or with instruments, **tying three knots** in alternating directions. Tie with enough tension to gently **evert** the wound, as this position enables optimal healing.
- **Cut** the thread, being sure to leave enough to enable easy removal at a later date.
- **Repeat** the process, spacing the remaining sutures evenly along the wound.
- Apply a **sterile dressing**.
- **Safely dispose** of sharps in a clinical sharps bin.
- **Dispose** of waste in clinical waste bins, and clean tray.
- Remove gloves, and **wash hands**.
- Thank the patient, and ensure that they are comfortable and have no adverse effects. Advise the patient of an approximate date of **suture removal** if non-absorbable sutures have been used, of the **signs of inflammation** to be aware of and to seek medical attention if they are noticed.
- **Record** in the **patient notes** the time, date, signature, name, designation and any difficulties that were encountered.

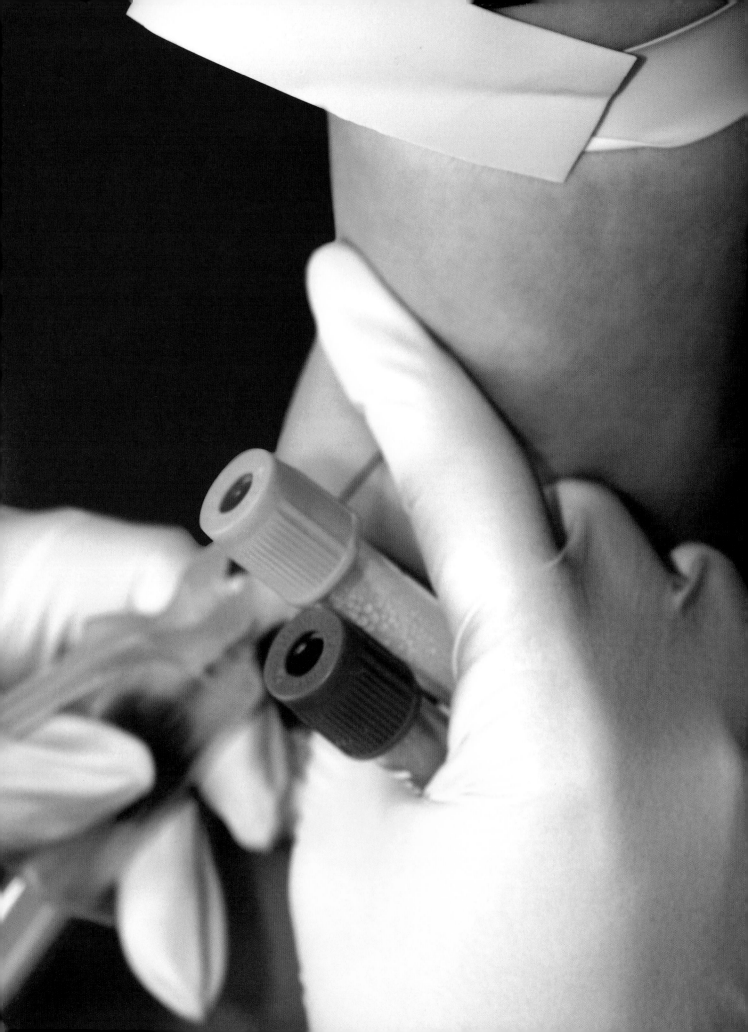

Administering medications

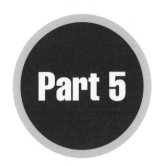

Part 5

Chapters

16 Administering intravenous infusions 40
17 Administering intravenous infusions of blood and
    blood products 42
18 Administering parenteral medications 44
19 Administering injections 46

16 Administering intravenous infusions

Figure 16.1 Colloid and crystalloid giving sets

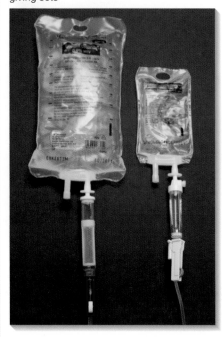

Figure 16.2 Administration of intravenous infusion with a pump

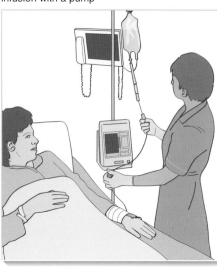

Hints and tips:

- Always **flush** a cannula with normal saline prior to use.
- Ask a **colleague** to check all **names**, **dates** and **doses** prior to administration.
- There are **two types** of infusion sets – colloid (for e.g. Gelofusin® or blood) and crystalloid (for e.g. normal saline or 5% dextrose). **Infusion pumps** have **dedicated sets**. Ensure you use the correct one!
- Remember to **clean** the bung prior to connection.
- Ensure you evaluate the patient's **cardiovascular system**.
- Ensure you evaluate the patient's **fluid status**.

Figure 16.3 Intravenous infusion prescription on dedicated region of medication card

Infusions

| Date & Time | Infusion Solution | | | | Medicine Added | | Prescriber | | | Administration | | | | Given by | Pharm |
	Type	Volume	Route	Rate	Approved name	Dose	Signature	Print name	Bleep	Date	Start Time	Stop Time	Vol. Given	Checked by	
2/10 0800	0.9 % SALINE	1L	IV	8"	KCl	20mmol	R Thomas	RACHEL THOMAS	#426	2/10	1000	1800	1L	JR LP	BW
2/10 0800	5% GLUCOSE	1L	IV	8"	–	–	R Thomas	RACHEL THOMAS	#426						

Figure 16.4 Equipment for an IV infusion

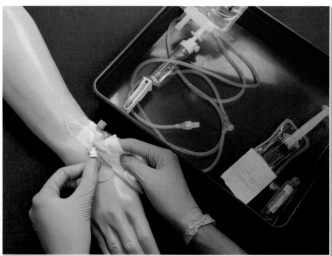

Figure 16.5 Roll the wheel clamp closed prior to use

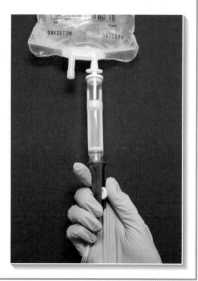

Practical Medical Procedures at a Glance, First Edition. Rachel K. Thomas © Rachel K. Thomas. Published 2015 by John Wiley & Sons, Ltd.
Companion website: http://www.ataglanceseries.com/practicalmedprocedures

What is an intravenous infusion?

An **intravenous (IV) infusion** is fluid administered **directly** into the **patient's vein**. This is usually done via a **cannula** (see Chapter 13) and a **giving set** (Figure 16.1). Fluid is run through the entire length of the giving set (also known as 'priming the line') **to remove any air bubbles** in the line, prior to actually administering the fluid. The administration of an IV infusion is a **daily occurrence** in any hospital and is frequently performed by nursing staff. In **emergencies**, however, you may be required to set up and administer them.

Infusions increase the **volume** of fluid in the patient's circulation, and therefore their **cardiovascular system** and their **fluid status** should be assessed prior to IV infusion administration. **Clinical requirements** must be weighed against **comorbidities** and **physiological parameters**, such as renal failure, heart failure, liver failure, dehydration or fluid overload, to determine the appropriate **rate** and **volume** for each clinical scenario, and these should be **documented** in the patient's notes.

Why are intravenous infusions important?

IV infusions are done for various reasons, such as in cases where maintenance fluid is required due to **inadequate oral intake** or **increased excretion** causing **dehydration**, or where a **quick delivery** is required – for example, when a patient is hypotensive due to sepsis.

It can be used in situations where other delivery methods may lead to more **side effects**, or if **other routes** of delivery are not appropriate. For instance, some medications such as chemotherapy may be given by infusion.

It may also be used if a **closely monitored level** of a medication is required, particularly if the medication has a narrow therapeutic window – for instance, heparin and insulin infusions.

A **pump** may also be used (Figure 16.2). These help to maintain a **steady delivery** of the fluid or medication over a specified timeframe, and are usually programmed by nursing staff depending on hospital protocols, according to the rate specified in the prescription.

Intravenous infusions must be **prescribed**, and within the prescription, the **rate** must be specified (Figure 16.3, and see Chapter 10). There are different types of commonly used fluids which require **different giving sets** – crystalloids (e.g. normal saline, 5% dextrose, dextrose–saline and Hartmann's or Lactated Ringer's solutions) and **colloids** (e.g. Gelofusine®, blood and blood products such as human albumin).

Indications

- Administration of IV fluids for maintenance, dehydration, poor oral intake, hypovolaemia
- Administration of medication
- Administration of blood and other products

Contra-indications

- Allergy
- Patient refusal

Complications

- **Local** – tissuing, infection
- **Systemic** – infection, allergy, electrolyte imbalances, fluid overload

Did you know?

- Best practice is for fluids to be infused through an infusion **pump**.
- Gravity infusion: in a **standard giving set**, 20 drops = 1 ml. This is usually specified on the back of the giving set. To calculate the drip rate:

$$ml/hr \times number\ of\ drops/ml\ of\ giving\ set / 60\ min = drops/min$$

Manually count the drops, and adjust the roller clamp over a minute.

Procedure

- Ensure that the IV fluid has been **prescribed** (Figure 16.3, and see Chapter 10).
- Ensure that the patient has a **cannula** inserted. If not, insert one (see Chapter 13).
- **Introduce** yourself, and **identify** the patient (see Chapter 4).
- Gain **consent** for the procedure (see Chapter 5), explain **indications** and check for **contra-indications** or **allergies**.
- Ensure **bare below the elbows**, and **wash hands** (see Chapter 6).
- Wipe clean a **tray** with antibacterial wipes.
- Collect equipment (Figure 16.4) and place it in a tray using the **aseptic non-touch technique (ANTT)** (see Chapter 8), including:
  - Non-sterile gloves
  - Chlorhexidine wipes
  - IV infusion giving set
  - IV fluid bag for infusion
  - Saline flush (see Chapter 13).
- **Check** the **expiry date** of the prescribed fluid.
- **Remove packaging** of the prescribed fluid, and **remove port cover**, taking care to **not touch the key part**.
- **Remove packaging** of the giving set, and **turn roller/wheel clamp off** (Figure 16.5).
- **Insert** the **sharp end** of the **giving set (spike)** into the **port of the IV fluid bag**, taking care to **not touch the key parts**.
- **Hang** the **fluid bag** on the **drip stand**.
- **Squeeze the drip** chamber until it is half filled with fluid.
- **Open** the giving set by rolling the **roller/wheel clamp open**, and run fluid through the **entire length** of the tubing so that **no air** remains in the line. (**Prime the line of the giving set.**)
- **Close** the giving set by rolling the **roller/wheel clamp closed** (Figure 16.5).
- **Hang giving set over drip stand**, or attach to **roller/wheel clamp** to help reduce contamination.
- **Wash hands**, and put on **gloves**.
- **Clean** the edge of the **bung** of the patient's cannula with a **chlorhexidine wipe**, and allow to dry for 30 seconds.
- **Flush** the cannula, if not newly inserted (see Chapter 13).
- Remove the cap of the giving set, and **attach to the needle-free bung** of the cannula, using **ANTT** and thus ensuring that **key parts** are not touched (see Chapter 8).
- **Open** the giving set by rolling the **roller/wheel clamp open**, check that the infusion runs freely when fully opened and then adjust the drip rate according to the prescription. Remove gloves, and **wash hands**.
- **Document** in the **patient notes**, including date, time, designation, contact details and any **problems** that may have been encountered.
- **Document** on the **fluid chart**, including the batch number of fluid, start time, and pump number if one is used.
- Dispose of waste in clinical waste bins, and clean tray.
- **Thank patient**, and ensure that they are comfortable and have no adverse effects.
- Ensure that the patient is **monitored** whilst the infusion is given. Continue with **vital sign** measurements, and include specific monitoring if this is required.

17 Administering intravenous infusions of blood and blood products

Figure 17.1 Blood type compatibilities

	Donor							
Type	O–	O+	B–	B+	A–	A+	AB–	AB+
AB+	✓	✓	✓	✓	✓	✓	✓	✓
AB–	✓		✓		✓		✓	
A+	✓	✓			✓	✓		
A–	✓				✓			
B+	✓	✓	✓	✓				
B–	✓		✓					
O+	✓	✓						
O–	✓							

(Recipient shown along left vertical axis)

Figure 17.2 Example of a blood bag

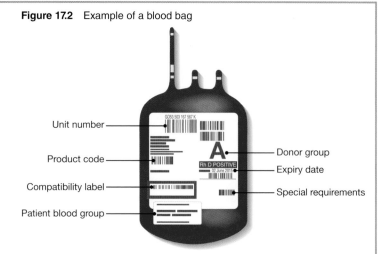

Unit number

Product code

Compatibility label

Patient blood group

Donor group

Expiry date

Special requirements

Figure 17.3 Intravenous infusion prescription on dedicated region of medication card

Blood transfusions

Date & Time	Infusion Solution			Prescriber			Administration				Given by / Checked by	Unit/Batch No.	Pharm
	Type	Volume	Rate	Signature	Print name	Bleep	Date	Start Time	Stop Time	Vol. Given			
2/10 1830	RED BLOOD CELLS	1 UNIT	4°	R Thomas	RACHEL THOMAS	#426	2/10	1830	2230	1L	LP / HR	EL9207164	BW

Hints and tips:

- Ensure you evaluate the patient's **cardiovascular system**.
- Ensure you evaluate the patient's **fluid status**.
- Ensure **regular monitoring** of the patient and their vital signs while the blood is being given and afterwards as clinically indicated.
- Insert a **large-bore cannula** if the uid needs to be given **quickly**.
- **Diuretic cover** may be required for some patients if the infusion may uid-overload them.
- **Flush** the cannula with saline after the transfusion.

Figure 17.4
A blood-giving set, showing mesh to filter out thrombi (large circle), and key parts (two smaller circles)

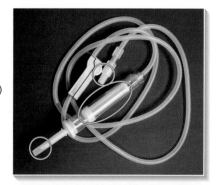

Did you know?

Transfusion reactions include:
- **Haemolytic transfusion reaction** – signs of hypotension, tachycardia, significantly raised temperature
- **Non-haemolytic transfusion reaction** – slightly raised temperature
- **Fluid overload** – shortness of breath, tachycardia, decreased oxygen saturation
- **Allergy** – itching, urticaria
- **Anaphylaxis** – swelling, hypotension, cyanosis, tachycardia, shortness of breath, decreased oxygen saturation

Figure 17.5
Transfusion of blood

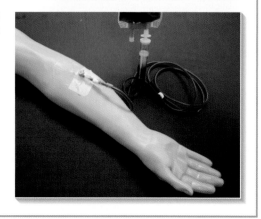

Practical Medical Procedures at a Glance, First Edition. Rachel K. Thomas © Rachel K. Thomas. Published 2015 by John Wiley & Sons, Ltd.
Companion website: http://www.ataglanceseries.com/practicalmedprocedures

What is an intravenous infusion of blood or blood products?

This is when **blood components** (or, less commonly, **whole blood**) are administered to a patient **directly into their veins**. Blood products that are transfused include **packed red cells, platelets, fresh frozen plasma, cryoprecipitate** and **human albumin**.

Prior to administration, the patient's blood group is determined, and it is **cross-matched** to determine the patient's antibodies. O-negative blood is the '**universal donor**', as all blood groups can receive this type of blood safely and this is used in emergencies or where the patient has not yet been matched (Figures 17.1 and 17.2).

As these infusions increase the patient's circulating volume, it is important to carry out a full clinical examination, including an assessment of the patient's **cardiovascular system, renal function** and **fluid status**, prior to intravenous (IV) administration. For example, a patient with heart failure or kidney disease may need a slower delivery **rate** and smaller **volume**, to avoid fluid overload and pulmonary oedema. This assessment is beyond the scope of this book, but it is important, and it needs to be **documented** in the patient notes.

Why are blood and blood product infusions important?

Various clinical conditions require transfusions for **treatment**. **Anaemia**, whether severe or symptomatic, may require red blood cells to be transfused. Generally, transfusing **1 unit** of red blood cells raises the haemoglobin by **1g/dL**. **Deranged clotting** may require platelets, fresh frozen plasma or cryoprecipitate. Whole blood may be used in **exchange transfusions**. **Human albumin** may be used in some cases of low protein levels.

Certain blood products only stay viable for a specific **time**. This will vary with local protocols, but, for example, red blood cells must be given within 4 hours of them reaching the ward, platelets are viable for 5 days, whilst fresh frozen plasma or cryoprecipitate may last for many months. Some Healthcare Trusts do not perform **non-emergency** transfusions during out-of-hours times, as there is an increased risk of error. Ensure that you become familiar with local protocols.

Some patients may **refuse** blood products for various reasons – for instance, Jehovah's Witnesses may refuse them on religious grounds. In such cases, check with a senior; however, if the patient has capacity (see Chapter 5), they are able to refuse such a treatment. Ensure that any such cases are **documented** fully and clearly in the notes.

Indications
- Anaemia (Hb <8 g/dL) or haemorrhage – red blood cells
- Severely deranged clotting – fresh frozen plasma, platelets, cryoprecipitate

Contra-indications
- Patient refusal
- Overloaded fluid status

Complications
- **Local** – allergic reaction, urticaria
- **Systemic** – anaphylaxis, fluid overload, non-haemolytic and haemolytic transfusion reactions

Procedure

Prior to commencing, **request** and **receive** the blood or blood components via local hospital protocols. These differ significantly in different areas; however, they usually involve both a **formal written request** and a **telephone confirmation request**, in order for the blood or blood products to be delivered. Ensure that this is performed and that the blood is ready prior to commencing the procedure given below.

- Ensure that the blood or blood components have been **prescribed** (Figure 17.3, and see Chapter 10).
- **Introduce** yourself, and **identify** the patient (see Chapter 4).
- Gain **consent** for the procedure (see Chapter 5), explain **indications** and check for **contra-indications** or **allergies**.
- Ensure **bare below the elbows**, and **wash hands** (see Chapter 6).
- Check for any previous **transfusions and transfusion reactions**.
- Take a **blood sample**, using the **venepuncture** technique (see Chapter 11) for **group and save** and/or **cross match**.
- Insert a **cannula** if one is not present, using the **cannulation** technique. A sample may be obtained from the cannula (see Chapter 13).
- Set up **IV infusion**, using the IV infusion technique (see Chapter 16). Use a **blood-giving set** or colloid-giving set (see Figure 17.4). This has an **in-line filter**.
- **Prime the line** of the giving set with **normal saline**, to ensure that there is **no air in the line** (see Chapter 16).
- **Wash hands**, and put on **gloves**.
- **Check** the **expiry date** and **identification details** on the blood or blood products **with the patient** and **with a colleague** prior to connection, **at the bedside**.
- **Connect** the blood-giving set to the cannula using the **aseptic non-touch technique (ANTT)** and thus not touching **key parts** (see Chapter 8).
- **Replace the saline with the blood product**.
- Roll open the clasp on the giving set so that the transfusion can begin, and specify the rate as required (Figure 17.5).
- Dispose of waste in clinical waste bins, and clean tray.
- Remove gloves, and **wash hands**.
- **Thank patient**, and ensure that they are comfortable and have no adverse effects.
- **Document** in the **patient notes** that patient has given **informed consent** and that the blood has been **prescribed** and **given**, including date, time, designation, contact details and any **problems** that may have been encountered.
- Ensure that the patient is **monitored** whilst the blood is being given for signs of **transfusion reaction, anaphylaxis** and **fluid overload**. **Vital signs** should be monitored frequently, such as every 15 minutes (see Chapter 9).

18 Administering parenteral medications

Figure 18.1 Glass ampoules of medications

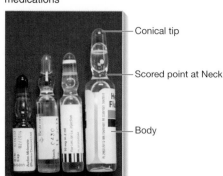

- Conical tip
- Scored point at Neck
- Body

Figure 18.2 Carefully snap at the neck

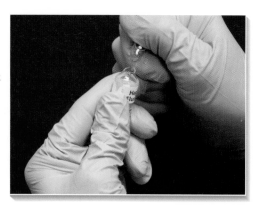

Figure 18.3 Carefully mixing and drawing up the medication

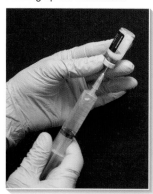

Figure 18.4 Intravenous medication prescribed on the medication card

Once Only Medications

Date	Time	Medication	Dose	Route	Signature	Given			Pharmacy
						Date	Time	Initials	
3/2/15	1445	FUROSEMIDE	40 mg	IV	R Thomas	3/2/15	1500	AK	LWC

Figure 18.5 Equipment tray, including two saline flushes and medication

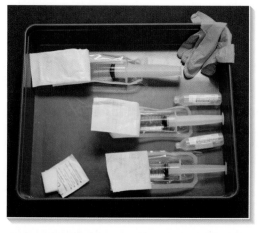

Figure 18.6 Intravenous administration of a medication

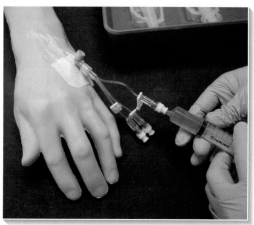

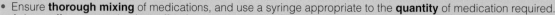

Hints and tips:

- Ensure **thorough mixing** of medications, and use a syringe appropriate to the **quantity** of medication required.
- Ask a **colleague** to check **medication name, expiry date** and **dose** – Remember: **doses vary** according to their route of administration.
- **Always** use a **fine-gauge needle** to draw up medications, to ensure any small pieces of glass are not injected.
- **Flush** with **normal saline before** and **after** administration – before to ensure the cannula is sited correctly with no swelling or pain, and after to ensure all of the medication is administered into the circulation (and not sitting in the cannula!).
- Ensure **air bubbles** are **removed** prior to administration – draw up more medication than prescribed, so that if some is discarded during bubble removal, the full dose is still available in the syringe.

What is parenteral administration?

Parenteral administration of medication is the administration of medication via any route that is not enteral (via the gut). This includes routes such as the **intravenous (IV)** administration of medications, directly into the patient's **vein** with a **syringe** or **infusion** via a **cannula** (see Chapter 13). This generally requires

two practitioners, as the medications need to be checked prior to administration. Other routes of administration are intramuscular, subcutaneous and intradermal (see Chapter 19).

Drugs are packaged as a **liquid**, in a vial or ampoule (Figures 18.1 and 18.2), or as a powder which requires **mixing** and **reconstitution** (Figure 18.3). The powder is mixed with **saline**, **water** or

Practical Medical Procedures at a Glance, First Edition. Rachel K. Thomas © Rachel K. Thomas. Published 2015 by John Wiley & Sons, Ltd.
Companion website: http://www.ataglanceseries.com/practicalmedprocedures

dextrose as a **diluent** for injection as per the specific medication's instructions, which are known as **monographs**. Instructions for reconstitution and administration can be found in local **hospital protocols and guidelines** (pharmacy sites) and fully explained in resources such as the **British National Formulary (BNF)**. As with any medications, parenteral medications must be **prescribed** on the medication card, and **allergies**, **contra-indications**, **interactions** and all other aspects relating to the safe prescription of medications need to be considered (Figure 18.4, and see Chapter 10).

Why are parenteral medications important?

Parenteral administration may be used when a **sustained** and **monitored** delivery is required, such as in insulin sliding scales or inotropes. In these cases, ensure that the medications are **thoroughly mixed** so that an accurate and predictable amount is delivered, and ensure that adequate **monitoring** is instituted.

Parenteral administration may also be used when other routes are **not appropriate**. For instance, a patient with significant nausea and vomiting may not tolerate anti-emetics orally, and an IV route may be appropriate. Various antibiotics may be given via this route, particularly when **fast delivery** and **absorption** are required. For instance, a patient may require IV morphine postoperatively if their pain is not adequately managed with other analgesia, or an IV injection of calcium gluconate may be required if a patient's potassium is raised.

Delivery via a cannula enables the medications to be delivered to the patient **without multiple injections**, as the cannula may remain *in situ* for several days (see Chapter 13).

Indications
- Administration of medications when other routes are not appropriate, or when fast absorption or sustained delivery is required

Contra-indications
- Allergy
- Patient refusal

Complications
- **Local** – phlebitis
- **Systemic** – infection, anaphylaxis, overdose

Procedure
- **Introduce** yourself, and **identify** the patient (see Chapter 4).
- Gain **consent** (see Chapter 5), explain **indications** and check for **contra-indications** or **allergies**.
- **Check** the **prescription** for dose, medication, route and time (Figure 18.4, and see Chapter 10).
- Check patient **allergies** and medication **name, dose** and **expiry date** with a colleague.
- Ensure **bare below the elbows**, and **wash hands** (see Chapter 6).
- Wipe clean a **tray** with antibacterial wipes.
- Collect equipment (Figure 18.5) and place in the tray using the **aseptic non-touch technique (ANTT)** (see Chapter 8), including:
  - Non-sterile gloves
  - Medication and prescription
  - 2× saline flushes, labelled (see Chapter 13)
  - Syringe of appropriate size for the quantity of medication required
  - Drawing-up needle
  - Medication ampoule, and fluid for reconstitution if required
  - Chlorhexidine wipes.

For medications not requiring mixing:
- **Wash hands**, and put on **gloves** (Health and Safety requirement, Control of Substances Hazardous to Health Regulations 2002; see Chapter 6).
- Label the syringe check prescription and sign.
- **Snap open medication ampoule** (Figure 18.2).
- **Attach drawing-up needle** to syringe, ensuring that no key parts are touched, using **ANTT** (see Chapter 8).
- **Insert** needle into ampoule, **invert**, and **draw back** on the syringe plunger to obtain the prescribed quantity of medication.
- **Remove air bubbles** (see Chapter 13).
- **Safely dispose** of **ampoule** and **needle** in clinical sharps bins.
- Place syringe back in its original packaging to protect **key part**.

For medications requiring mixing:
- **Wash hands**, and put on **gloves**.
- Check **name, expiry date** and **lot number** of diluent.
- Check **name, expiry date** and **lot number** of medication.
- Label the syringe with the above information, check prescription and sign.
- Attach **drawing-up needle** to the syringe, ensuring no key parts are touched, using **ANTT**, and draw up **diluent** as though preparing a flush (see Chapter 13). Dispose of needle in the sharps container.
- Change needles.
- Remove plastic lid (dust cap), if present, and **wipe cap** of vial with a chlorhexidine wipe. Allow to dry for 30 seconds.
- **Insert needle** into **dedicated region** on cap, and **inject** correct quantity of **diluent** into the vial to dissolve the powdered drug (see Figure 18.3).
- **Thoroughly mix** the solution.
- **Draw back** on syringe to obtain the required quantity of reconstituted medication, and **remove air bubbles** (see Chapter 19).
- **Safely dispose** of **vial** and **needle** in clinical sharps bins.
- Place syringe back in its original packaging to protect **key part**.

For all parenteral medications:
- **RECHECK IDENTITY, PRESCRIPTION and ALLERGIES**
- Clean **cannula needle-free bung** with a chlorhexidine wipe, and **do not touch this key part**.
- To ensure cannula is sited accurately, **flush cannula** with saline by inserting the nozzle of the saline-filled syringe into the end of the cannula, **not touching key parts**, and slowly depressing plunger (see Chapter 13). **Inspect** for swelling or pain.
- Attach syringe to cannula using **ANNT**, taking care to not touch **key parts**.
- **Administer** the medication slowly (Figure 18.6), usually over a few minutes (according to the monograph), observing for adverse reactions.
- **Dispose of syringe** in a clinical waste bin.
- **Clean bung** with a chlorhexidine wipe; do not touch this **key part**, and **flush it again** with saline.
- **Dispose** of waste in clinical waste bins, and wipe tray clean.
- Remove gloves, and **wash hands**.
- **Record** in the **patient notes** time, date, signature, name, designation and **lot number** of medication used, and any difficulties encountered.
- **Record** in **medication card** the **time** the dose was given.
- **Thank patient**, and ensure that they are comfortable and have no adverse effects.
- Ensure appropriate **monitoring** is in place.

19 Administering injections

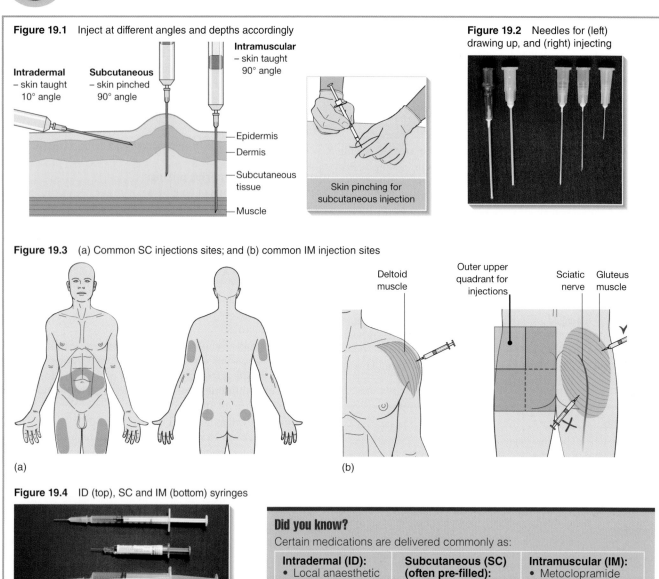

Figure 19.1 Inject at different angles and depths accordingly

Intradermal
– skin taught
10° angle

Subcutaneous
– skin pinched
90° angle

Intramuscular
– skin taught
90° angle

Epidermis
Dermis
Subcutaneous tissue
Muscle

Skin pinching for subcutaneous injection

Figure 19.2 Needles for (left) drawing up, and (right) injecting

Figure 19.3 (a) Common SC injections sites; and (b) common IM injection sites

(a)

(b)

Deltoid muscle

Outer upper quadrant for injections

Sciatic nerve

Gluteus muscle

Figure 19.4 ID (top), SC and IM (bottom) syringes

Did you know?
Certain medications are delivered commonly as:

Intradermal (ID):	Subcutaneous (SC) (often pre-filled):	Intramuscular (IM):
• Local anaesthetic	• Heparin	• Metoclopramide
• Allergy testing	• Insulin	• Haloperidol

What are the types of injections?

Injections are named according to the tissue into which they are administered (Figure 19.1). Different layers cause different degrees of drug release, with **intradermal (ID)** injections remaining **localised**, while **subcutaneous (SC)**, **intramuscular (IM)** and **intravenous (IV)** injections are used to achieve different objectives that are dependent on the clinically required absorption.

Injections are significantly less painful for the patient if a good technique is developed and practised. Different types of needles are used for the different injections (Figure 19.2); however, the type used also depends on clinical factors such as body habitus.

Why are the types of injections important?

Different injections are important for delivering **different medications** at **different rates**.

ID injections are used for very **localised administration** of medications. They are most commonly used for **local anaesthetic,** for example prior to an arterial blood gas measurement to minimise pain (now as part of the British Thoracic Society guidelines). Ensure the strength of the medication is checked prior to administration, particularly with local anaesthetics. **Avoid** injection of local anaesthetic–adrenaline mixtures in peripheral structures, as there is a risk of inducing ischaemia. ID injections are also commonly used for **allergy testing**.

SC injections are used to administer drugs delivered systemically at a **slower absorption rate**. Common injection sites for SC injections include the **arm**, **thigh**, **abdomen** and **buttock** (Figure 19.3a). It may be appropriate to **vary** the site if repeated injections are to be administered, as in the case of insulin and heparin.

IM injections are used to deliver **large, quick-acting doses** as muscles have a good blood supply. These may be **painful**. This is

Practical Medical Procedures at a Glance, First Edition. Rachel K. Thomas © Rachel K. Thomas. Published 2015 by John Wiley & Sons, Ltd.
Companion website: http://www.ataglanceseries.com/practicalmedprocedures

due to the fact that a relatively large volume is squeezed into a muscle that has no space to accommodate it. Various sites are possible for this type of injection. Commonly sites are the **deltoid**, **anterior midthigh** and **ventro-gluteal region** (Figure 19.3b). SC and IM injections should be injected at a rate of **1 ml every 10 seconds**.

Indications
- Various, dependent upon the medication requirements and speed of administration

Contra-indications
- Infection at site
- Patient refusal or allergy
- Bleeding disorder

Complications
- **Local** – pain or bruising at site, haematoma, fat necrosis
- **Systemic** – anaphylaxis

Hints and tips:
- Always adhere to **local protocols** where available.
- **Needle sizes** may need to be adjusted for **obese** or **emaciated** patients.
- To expel an air bubble, gently tap the side of the syringe whilst gently pushing up the plunger.
- Remember to **aspirate** prior to injecting.
- **Wait** several seconds before withdrawing the needle, to ensure the medication has been delivered.
- **Vary injection** sites for repeated doses.

Procedure

Introduce yourself, and **identify** the patient (see Chapter 4).
- Gain **consent** for the procedure (see Chapter 5), explain **indications** and check for **contra-indications** or **allergies**.
- **Check** the **prescription** for dose, medication, route and time (see Chapter 10).
- Ensure **bare below the elbows**, and **wash hands** (see Chapter 6).
- Wipe clean a **tray** with antibacterial wipes.
- Collect equipment and place in the tray using the **aseptic non-touch technique (ANTT)** (see Chapter 8), including:
  - Prescription
  - Non-sterile gloves
  - Gauze and tape
  - Pre-filled syringe of medication, or all of the following:
    - Prescribed medication
    - Syringe of appropriate size for the quantity of medication required
    - Needle
    - Drawing-up needle.
- Check **medication name**, **expiry date** and **lot number**.
- **Wash hands**, and put on **gloves** (Health and Safety requirement, Control of Substances Hazardous to Health Regulations 2002; see Chapter 6).
- Attach **drawing-up needle** to **syringe**, using **ANTT** and thus **not touching key parts**.
- Draw up medication (see Chapter 18). If medication has a cap, wipe lid clean using a chlorhexidine wipe.
- Label the syringe.
- **Safely dispose** of drawing-up needle in clinical sharps bins, and replace with appropriate-gauge needle using **ANTT** and thus **not touching key parts** (Figures 19.2 and 19.4).
  ID – fine-gauge needle (orange hub 25G)
  SC – often pre-packaged, or fine-gauge needle (orange hub 25G)
  IM – larger gauge needle (green hub 21G or blue hub 23G).

- Place in tray, remove gloves and wash hands.
- Move to patient, if setup was in a different area.
- **Wash hands**, and put on **gloves** (not a World Health Organization requirement).
- **Select injection site** (Figure 19.3a and 19.3b):
  ID – as clinically indicated, preferably not at extremities for local anaesthetic
  SC – commonly arm, thigh, abdomen or buttock
  IM – commonly deltoid, quadriceps or gluteals.
- **Clean** injection site, or ensure site is socially clean (according to local policy).
- Warn patient of a **sharp scratch.**
- Insert needle with the **bevel up** (Figure 19.1).
  ID – at a shallow angle, approximately **10°**, just below the epidermal layer.
  SC – may bunch up the patient's skin, so only adipose tissue is held or you may pull skin taut and inject at a **90° angle**.
  IM – pull skin taut, inject perpendicular to the skin surface and insert needle at a **90° angle**.
- **Aspirate**, by pulling back on the plunger, prior to injection to ensure needle is not in a blood vessel.
- **Inject medication slowly** (SC and IM at **1 ml every 10 seconds**, or until a wheal or **bleb** of prescribed dose occurs in ID).
- **Wait before withdrawing**, approximately 5–10 seconds.
- **Withdraw** and dispose of all waste, and **safely dispose** of sharps in clinical sharps bin.
- Thank the patient, ensure they are comfortable and have no adverse effects and apply a dressing over the puncture site.
- Remove gloves, and **wash hands**.
- **Record** in the notes **time**, **date**, **signature**, **name**, **designation** and medication **lot number** and any difficulties encountered.
- Continue appropriately with the next procedure if required, including **monitoring** of clotting if heparin is administered, and blood glucose levels if insulin is administered.

Aspects of injecting

Select a syringe of **suitable size**, with **suitable markings** to enable accurate drug delivery for each specific case – for instance, some syringes are marked at 0.2 ml, whilst others are at 1 ml. Always ensure that the **medication's name**, **expiry date** and **lot number** are checked prior to administration. All syringes must be appropriately **labelled**. Have a **colleague** also confirm this with you prior to injection. As with all medications and interventions, remember to correctly identify the patient and any **allergies** that they may have, prior to administration.

Needles are also referred to as **hypodermic** needles, as they are used to administer medications under (hence *hypo*) the skin (hence, *dermic*). They are different diameters, referred to as gauge (Figure 19.2). A **larger diameter needle** will have a **smaller gauge number**. For instance, the larger diameter 21G needle is used for IM injections, whilst a smaller diameter 25G needle is used for ID injections. These needle sizes need to be adjusted for each patient as clinically indicated – an obese patient may require a different needle compared to one who is emaciated or cachectic.

Once the needle has been inserted, immediately prior to injecting the medication, ensure that you pull back on the plunger slightly. This is known as **aspirating**. If the needle is in a blood vessel, aspiration will reveal blood – in which case, withdraw the needle and start afresh.

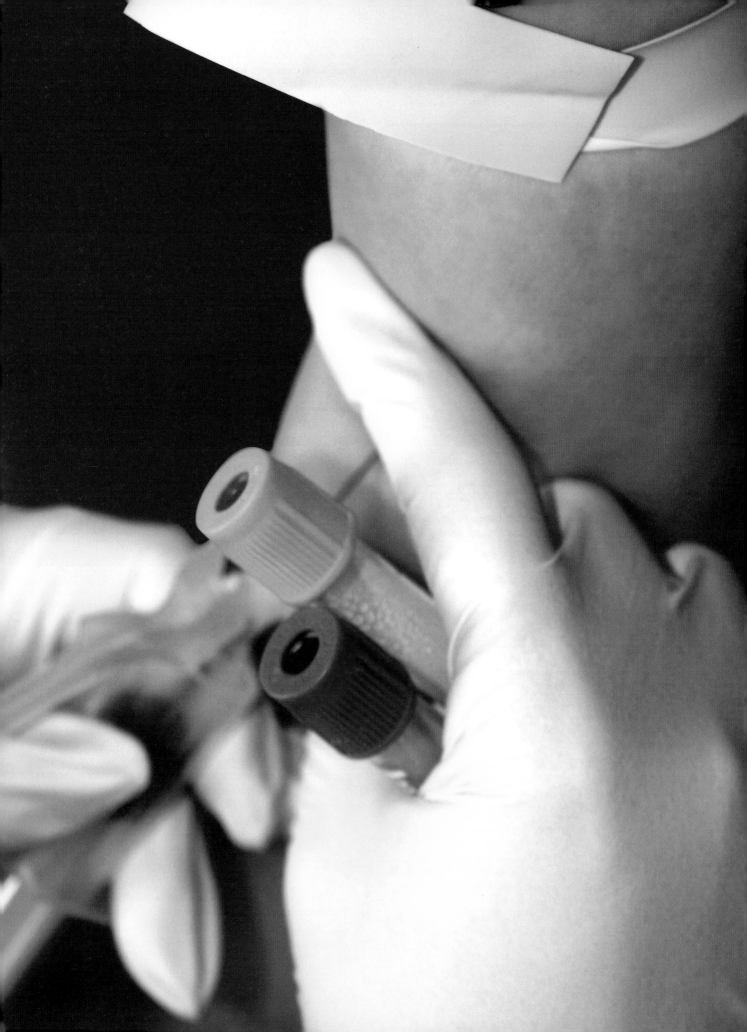

Common procedures – respiratory

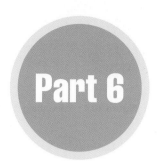

Part 6

Chapters

20 **Measuring arterial blood gas** 50
21 **Administering oxygen therapy** 52
22 **Using inhalers and nebulisers** 54
23 **Assessing respiratory function** 56
24 **Using airway manoeuvres and simple adjuncts** 58
25 **Ventilating with a bag valve mask device** 60

20 Measuring arterial blood gas

Figure 20.1 Performing the Modified Allen's test

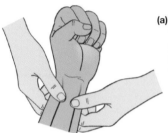

(a) Ask patient to clench fist tightly, apply enough pressure over the ulnar artery and the radial artery to collapse them

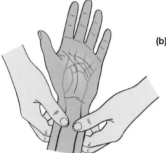

(b) Ask patient to open hand; the palm will be pale

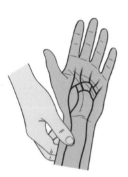

(c) Keep pressure over the radial artery, release pressure over the ulnar artery; palm will return to normal colour if the ulnar artery patent

Modified Allen's Test:

- This is done to ensure adequate patency of the ulnar artery, prior to taking a sample from the radial artery.
- Request the patient **clench fist tightly**.
- Using your fingers, find the **ulnar** and **radial arteries**.
- **Occlude** both arteries with pressure obstructing blood flow to the hand.
- Request the patient **relax their hand** and observe that palm is **pale**.
- **Release** the **ulnar artery**, and the hand should become **re-perfused** and **red** in less than 10 seconds, showing that this artery has good patency and flow. This flushing is **normal**, a positive modified Allen Test.
- If the hand does **not re-perfuse**, the ulnar artery is not supplying adequate blood flow to the hand, and the radial artery **must not be used** for the arterial blood gas sampling.

Figure 20.2 A sample printout

```
At 37C
pH_____7.490
PaCO2_____42.3   mmHg
PaO2_____88    mmHg
HCO3_____32    mmol/L
BEecf_____9     mmol/L
sO2*_____97    %
    *calculated

FIO2_____:  100
Sample Type_:  ART

  24MAY15      11:25
```

Table 20.1 Normal ABG ranges

Normal ABG ranges	
pH	7.35–7.45
PaO_2	>10 kPa
$PaCO_2$	4.7–6.0 kPa
HCO_3	22–26 mmol/L

Figure 20.3 Equipment for taking an ABG

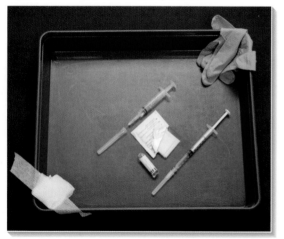

Figure 20.4 Normal site of ABG sampling

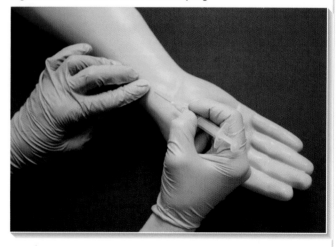

Practical Medical Procedures at a Glance, First Edition. Rachel K. Thomas © Rachel K. Thomas. Published 2015 by John Wiley & Sons, Ltd.
Companion website: http://www.ataglanceseries.com/practicalmedprocedures

What is an arterial blood gas?

An **arterial blood gas** (ABG) is a sample of blood taken directly from an **artery**. The artery most commonly used is the **radial artery** after ensuring the patency of the ulnar artery (Figure 20.1), but the femoral artery (or, less commonly, the brachial artery) can be used in emergency situations. The blood sample is collected in a **heparinised syringe** to prevent clotting prior to analysis. The sample is run through an **analyser**, producing a printout (Figure 20.2). Analysers are expensive, sophisticated equipment usually found in intensive care wards, emergency departments and paediatric, obstetric and respiratory wards.

Why is an ABG important?

An ABG sample can provide important information in diagnosis and management of patients in hospital. They enable results to be obtained **quickly**, rather than waiting for laboratory samples to be processed. Commonly, it is used to determine a patient's **respiratory** and **acid–base status** (i.e. **PaO_2, $PaCO_2$, pH, bicarbonate** and **base excess**; Table 20.1). The PaO_2, $PaCO_2$ and pH are **measured**, and all other values are **derived**. Modern blood gas analysers also measure haemoglobin, blood glucose, electrolytes and lactate which are very useful in the immediate assessment of the acutely unwell patient. They can also be used for **monitoring** patients and their therapy, such as whether patients with chronic obstructive pulmonary disorder are retaining carbon dioxide through over-enthusiastic use of oxygen therapy. In any patient, always ensure that the **patient's oxygen therapy concentration** (FiO_2) is recorded if they are being treated with supplemental oxygen.

Indications
- Respiratory disease
- Acutely or chronically unwell patient

Contra-indications
- Patient refusal
- Poor modified Allen's test result
- Arteriovenous fistula

Complications
- **Local** – pain, bruising, haematoma, infection, ischaemia
- **Systemic** – infection

Procedure

- **Introduce** yourself, and **identify** the patient (see Chapter 4).
- Gain **consent** for the procedure (see Chapter 5), explain **indications** and check for **contra-indications** or **allergies**.
- Ensure **bare below the elbows**, and **wash hands** (see Chapter 6).
- Wipe clean a **tray** with antibacterial wipes.
- Collect equipment (Figure 20.3) and place in the tray using the **aseptic non-touch technique (ANTT)** (see Chapter 8), including:
  - Non-sterile gloves
  - 23G needle
  - Heparinised syringe: low resistance, self-filling
  - Chlorhexidine wipe
  - Swab
  - Syringe filled with local anaesthetic (see Chapter 19).
- Lay out equipment in tray with packages opened but **key parts untouched**, and **assemble syringe and needle** if local protocols do not provide a **pre-assembled kit**.
- Expose the patient's **non-dominant arm**.
- Perform **modified Allen's test** (Figure 20.1).
- Identify the **radial artery and its path along the forearm**.
- **Wash hands**, and put on **gloves**.
- **Dosiflex** the wrist to assist in access to the artery.
- Palpate the radial artery with two fingers, and lift the distal finger whilst maintaining light palpation with the proximal finger (non-dominant hand).
- **Clean** intended puncture area with chlorhexidine wipe. Do not re-palpate this area, as it is a **key site**; instead, palpate the artery several centimetres higher.
- **Perform an intradermal local anaesthetic injection** (see Chapter 19). This is effective within 1 to 2 minutes.
- Holding syringe like a pencil, with the bevel facing upwards, penetrate the artery at an angle of **30° or less** to the skin, using the proximal finger of the non-dominant hand as a guide. The syringe will fill automatically due to the pressure of the artery (Figure 20.4).
- Minimising movement of the needle, fill the syringe with **1–2 ml** of blood.
- Withdraw the needle, and place **pressure** over the puncture site for at least 3 to 5 minutes (longer if the patient is on warfarin).
- **Agitate** the sample in the syringe to prevent clotting, and **expel air bubbles** by slowly depressing the plunger and tapping the side of the syringe.
- **Safely dispose** of needle in clinical sharps bin.
- Cap the syringe.
- Dispose of clinical waste in clinical waste bin, and clean tray.
- Thank the patient, and ensure that they are comfortable and have no adverse effects.
- **Document** in the **patient notes**, including date, time, designation, contact details and any **problems** that may have been encountered.
- **Label** the syringe containing the **specimen**.
- Take the sample to be **analysed**, ensuring the patient is **appropriately supervised** while doing so.
- Remove gloves, and **wash hands**.
- **Record results**, and take appropriate actions.

Did you know?
Taking an **arterial blood gas** (ABG) sample can often be painful for the patient – studies showed that asthmatics and diabetics were delaying presentation to hospitals, which was attributed partly to avoiding having these painful samples taken. It is now part of the British Thoracic Guidelines that **local anaesthetic** be given prior to ABG sampling (see Chapter 19).

Aspects of blood gases

It is important to note that in many acute settings, a **venous blood gas (VBG)** will offer adequate information. While this will not indicate the patient's blood oxygenation level (PaO_2), other values obtained will be useful. In order to perform a VBG, the same procedure is followed as with an ABG but a venous sample is obtained.

The interpretation of blood gases is beyond the scope of the book, but it is important to master this.

21 Administering oxygen therapy

Figure 21.1 (a, b) Nasal cannulae. Source for (b): Ward *et al* (2010), Chapter 43, p. 94.

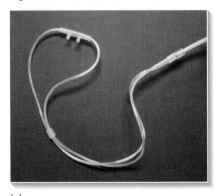

(a)

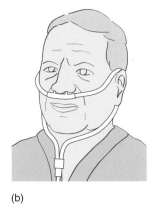

(b)

Figure 21.2 Simple oxygen face mask

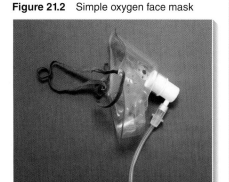

Figure 21.3 Venturi mask with adapters

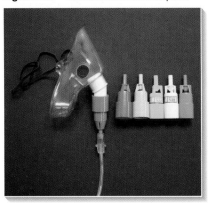

Figure 21.4 (a, b) Non-rebreathe mask. Source for (b): Ward *et al* (2010), Chapter 43, p. 94.

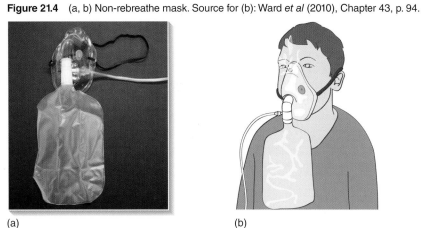

(a)

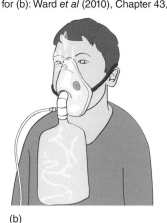

(b)

Figure 21.5 Oxygen prescription on a medication card

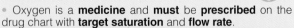

Oxygen

Month OCTOBER Date ⟶		2	3	4	5							
Oxygen												
Target Saturation: 88–92% (94–98%) Other:	0800	AK										
	1400	AK										
Flow rate: 2 L/min	1800											
(PRN) or Continous	2200											
Device: NASAL CANULAE												

Signature *K Thomas*	Print Name RACHEL THOMAS	Bleep #426	Comments

| Month   Date ⟶ | |

Hints and tips:

- Oxygen is a **medicine** and **must** be **prescribed** on the drug chart with **target saturation** and **flow rate**.
- In general, oxygen should be **gradually reduced** according to the patient's **tolerance**.
- Always check **arterial blood gases** in anyone at risk of **hypercapnic respiratory failure**.
- A **high oxygen requirement** is a sign of illness **severity** and may require frequent monitoring, ABG and senior input.

Table 21.1 Venturi adaptors and their corresponding flow rates

Type of Venturi (%)	Colour	Oxygen flow rate (L/min)
24	Blue	2–4
28	White	4–6
35	Yellow	8–10
40	Red	10–12
60	Green	12–14

Practical Medical Procedures at a Glance, First Edition. Rachel K. Thomas © Rachel K. Thomas. Published 2015 by John Wiley & Sons, Ltd.
Companion website: http://www.ataglanceseries.com/practicalmedprocedures

What is oxygen therapy?

Administering oxygen is key to managing patients who are **hypoxaemic** (oxygen saturations <94%). It is used in many acute and chronic medical conditions. There are several different devices for the administration of oxygen depending on the scenario. These include:

- **Nasal cannulae** (Figure 21.1a and 21.1b)
- **Simple oxygen face mask** (Figure 21.2)
- **Venturi mask** (Figure 21.3)
- **Non-rebreathe mask** (Figure 21.4a and 21.4b).

Oxygen must be **prescribed** on the **medication chart**, indicating the type of delivery device (Figure 21.5, and see Chapter 10). Each of the devices delivers oxygen at a different rate. **Nasal cannulae** are thin plastic tubes with two small nozzles that sit in the nostrils. They require 2 to 4 L/min and deliver 24–40% oxygen (variable). **Simple face masks** such as the Hudson mask deliver 24–60% oxygen and require 6 to 12 L/min. **Venturi masks** accurately deliver between 24% and 60% oxygen depending on the adapter used and the oxygen flow rate (Table 21.1). **Non-rebreathe masks** deliver the highest percentage of inspired oxygen (over 80%). A **bag-valve mask** is used if the patient is hypoventilating or no longer breathing spontaneously (apnoeic) (see Chapter 25).

Indications

- Emergency treatment
- Condition with hypoxaemia or respiratory disease

Contra-indications

- Patient refusal
- Evidence-based guidance where the use of oxygen may have no advantage (e.g. acute coronary syndrome and acute stroke)

Complications

- **Local** – discomfort
- **Systemic** – hypopnoea or apnoea in known CO_2 retainers where their hypoxic drive functions abnormally

Why is oxygen therapy important?

Hypoxaemia is present in **many conditions**, and it needs correcting to **optimise patient outcomes** – thus, oxygen is frequently prescribed. It may be due to a wide range of causes, from **respiratory disease** to **neurological disease**. It can be **acute** or **chronic**, but in all conditions, aiming for the appropriate oxygen saturations in the patient is a crucial part of their treatment. The target oxygen saturations of a healthy person are **94–98%**. In chronic obstructive pulmonary disease (COPD) and other conditions where there is a risk of hypercapnic respiratory failure, the target is **88–92%** (British Thoracic Society Guidance). **Target oxygen saturations must** be indicated on the **medication card** when oxygen is prescribed (see Figure 21.5).

It is important to note that a **high oxygen requirement** is a sign of illness **severity** and may require **frequent monitoring**, an **arterial blood gas** sample and **senior input**.

In **critical illness**, for example shock, sepsis and cardiac arrest, all patients should be given **high-flow oxygen** (15 L/min) via a **non-rebreathe mask** with target saturations of **94–98%**. If a patient is at risk of **hypercapnic respiratory failure**, they should still be started on high-flow oxygen with target saturations of 94–98% **pending results of ABGs** – the oxygen flow rate should be **adjusted** if the patient shows signs of **carbon dioxide retention**. In non-critical illness, patients at risk of carbon dioxide retention should be prescribed oxygen via a Venturi mask at **24–28%**.

Procedure

- **Introduce** yourself, and **identify** the patient (see Chapter 4).
- Gain **consent** for the procedure (see Chapter 5), explain **indications** and check for **contra-indications** or **allergies**.
- Ensure **bare below the elbows**, and **wash hands** (see Chapter 6).
- **Sit patient up**, and apply device, correctly indicating the appropriate flow rate as follows:
  - Nasal cannulae (2 L/min)
  - Venturi (according to device)
  - Simple face mask (5 to 10 L/min)
  - Non-rebreathe (12 to 15 L/min). Before applying the mask over the patient's face, **occlude the valve** at the opening of the reservoir bag to facilitate it filling with oxygen.
  - Apply **saturation probe**, and record reading (see Chapter 9).
  - **Prescribe** oxygen therapy on drug chart, sign and print name with contact details (Figure 21.5, and see Chapter 10).
  - **Adjust** oxygen therapy until saturations are within the target range (94–98% or 88–92%, as clinically appropriate), regularly **reviewed** and **adjusted**.
  - **Thank patient**, and ensure that they are comfortable and have no adverse effects.
  - **Wash hands**.

Did you know?

The desire to breathe is **normally** due to blood levels of **carbon dioxide**. In patients with chronically elevated levels, **desensitisation** occurs – they rely on blood levels of **oxygen** to drive their respiration. If the blood oxygen levels are artificially elevated, **hypoventilation** may result, thus increasing the risk of **hypercapnic respiratory failure**.

Aspects of oxygen therapy

Some patients with chronic hypoxaemia, nocturnal hypoventilation or palliative conditions may require oxygen in their own home; this is called **long-term oxygen therapy (LTOT)**. It must be administered for at least **15 hours/day** to improve survival. They should not smoke in order to be considered for this therapy, and they should have a PaO_2 of ≤7.3 or a PaO_2 of ≤8.0 with **additional risk factors** such as pulmonary hypertension.

For patients with **asthma**, nebulisers should be driven by **oxygen** at a flow rate of at least 6 L/min (see Chapter 22). Alternatively, an **air-driven** nebuliser can be used (and should be used for patients at risk of **hypercapnic respiratory failure**), with supplemental oxygen given via nasal cannulae at 2 to 6 L/min to maintain appropriate oxygen saturations.

22 Using inhalers and nebulisers

Figure 22.1 Aerosol metered dose inhaler

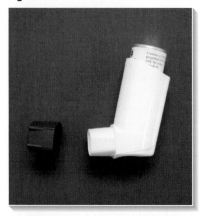

Figure 22.2 Breath-actuated inhaler

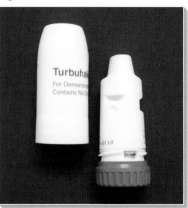

Figure 22.3 Dry powder inhaler

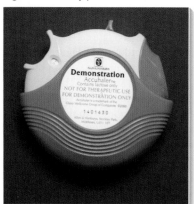

Figure 22.4 (a, b) Inhaler attached to spacer device

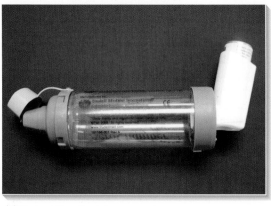

(a)

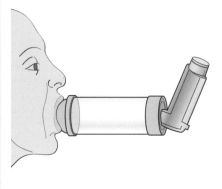

(b)

Figure 22.5 (a, b) Nebuliser kit. Source for (b): Davey (2014), Chapter 109, p. 243.

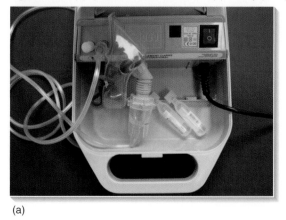

(a)

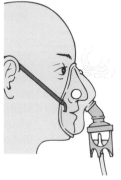

(b)

Did you know?

Inhalers may contain **more than one** inhaled drug:
- Seretide®: salmeterol and fluticasone
- Symbicort®: formoterol and budesonide
- Combivent®: salbutamol and ipratropium
- Fostair®: formoterol and beclometasone

What are inhalers and nebulisers?

Inhalers are small **handheld devices** used to **administer medications** (e.g. bronchodilators and steroids) to the airways in patients with **asthma** and **chronic obstructive pulmonary disorder (COPD)**. Types of **inhalers** available include:

- **Aerosol metered dose inhaler**, also known as a press-and-breathe pressurised metered dose inhaler (pMDI), **with or without a spacer** (Figures 22.1, 22.4a and 22.4b)
- **Breath-actuated inhalers** (Figure 22.2)
- **Dry powdered inhalers (DPIs)** (Figure 22.3).

Nebulisers can also be used to deliver medications into the airways (Figure 22.5a and 22.5b). A nebuliser passes either **oxygen** or **air** through an **aqueous solution** of a medicine, turning it into a **fine mist** which is **inhaled** by the patient. Inhalers and nebulisers need to be prescribed on the medication card, with the **route** listed as 'inhaled'.

Practical Medical Procedures at a Glance, First Edition. Rachel K. Thomas © Rachel K. Thomas. Published 2015 by John Wiley & Sons, Ltd.
Companion website: http://www.ataglanceseries.com/practicalmedprocedures

Why are inhalers and nebulisers important?

Both inhalers and nebulisers are used to deliver **inhaled medications** to the lungs. Both have **advantages** and **disadvantages**. Aerosol inhalers require the patient to **co-ordinate** inhalation with pressing down on the canister, which can be difficult, especially in the young and the elderly. Even with good technique, much of the drug is **deposited incorrectly** in the mouth and pharynx and does not reach the airways. If the inhaler is attached to a **spacer**, the co-ordination is easier (Figure 22.4). However, spacers are affected by **static charge**, and thus they need to be washed and wiped dry between uses. An advantage of breath-actuated and dry-powder devices is that the patient does not need to co-ordinate pressing down on the inhaler with timing of inhalation.

Nebulisers are mainly used for delivery of salbutamol and ipratropium in **acute asthma** and **COPD**. They are also used in lung conditions such as cystic fibrosis and bronchiectasis. Generally, a **mask** is used to deliver the medication, but a patient may also prefer to use a **handheld device** (Figure 22.5a). Nebulisers are required for **higher doses** of medication, when the medication cannot be delivered by another route or when the patient is **too unwell** to use another route.

Indications
- Diseases requiring medication to be delivered to the airways

Contra-indications
- Patient refusal
- Allergy to medication

Complications
- **Local** – discomfort
- **Systemic** – medication specific, for example anaphylaxis if there is an allergy, or tachycardia from salbutamol

Hints and tips:

- Patients **inhaling steroids** should **wash** their mouth out with water afterwards, to minimise the risk of candidiasis.
- **Check inhaler technique** if there is poor therapeutic response.
- Advise the patient to **wash** and **wipe dry spacers** in between use.

Procedure

For an **aerosol inhaler**:
- **Introduce** yourself, and **identify** the patient (see Chapter 4).
- Gain **consent** for the procedure (see Chapter 5), explain **indications** and check for **contra-indications** or **allergies**.
- Ensure **bare below the elbows**, and **wash hands** (see Chapter 6).
- Instruct patient to:
  - **Remove cap** and check that **mouthpiece** is clean.
  - **Shake** the inhaler and **breathe out** gently.
  - Place the mouthpiece in mouth and **seal with lips**.
  - **Breathe in** and **simultaneously** press canister.
  - Keep inhaler in mouth and **hold breath** for 10 seconds.
- **Repeat** the procedure after 30 to 60 seconds if required.

For an **aerosol inhaler with spacer device**:
- **Introduce** yourself, and **identify** the patient (see Chapter 4).
- Gain **consent** for the procedure (see Chapter 5), explain **indications** and check for **contra-indications** or **allergies**.
- Ensure **bare below the elbows**, and **wash hands** (see Chapter 6).
- Instruct patient to:
  - **Remove** cap and check that **mouthpiece** is clean.
  - **Shake** the inhaler and **insert into spacer**.
  - Place the mouthpiece of the spacer in the mouth and **seal with lips**.
  - **Breathe slowly out** to check the valve.
  - Press the canister of the inhaler, keeping the **spacer** in the mouth.
  - **Either** take a **slow deep breath**, hold for approximately 10 seconds and breathe out through the mouthpiece, **or breathe in and out** five times.
- Remove the device, and clean.
- **Repeat** after 30 to 60 seconds if a further dose is required.

For a **nebuliser**:
- **Introduce** yourself, and **identify** the patient (see Chapter 4).
- Gain **consent** for the procedure (see Chapter 5), explain **indications** and check for **contra-indications** or **allergies**.
- Ensure **bare below the elbows**, and **wash hands** (see Chapter 6).
- Collect equipment, including:
  - **Facemask** or **mouthpiece**
  - Nebuliser medication chamber
  - Compressor pack, power source or cylinder with driver gas (air or oxygen)
  - Medication to be administered.
- Check **medication** and **expiry date**.
- Deposit the prescribed amount of medications in the nebuliser chamber, which requires **4 to 10 ml**. Sodium chloride solution should be used to dilute the drugs, rather than water, unless stated.
- Assemble chamber, and connect to mask and driver source.
- Place the mask on patient's face, ensuring correct placement and flow rate (6 to 8 L/min).
- Delivery time should not be longer than **10 minutes** or device starts 'sputtering', after which the patient should be **re-assessed**.
- **Record** in the **patient notes** time, date, signature, name, designation and **lot number** of medication used, any difficulties encountered and the outcome of the medication.
- **Record** in medication card the **time** the dose was given.
- **Thank patient**, and ensure that they are comfortable and have no adverse effects.
- **Dispose** of waste in clinical waste bins.
- **Wash hands**.

Did you know?

Asthma symptoms include wheeze, cough (particularly at night-time), shortness of breath and chest tightness. **Inhaler therapy** starts with use of a '**reliever**' when symptoms present. A '**preventer**' is added, and used daily, if symptoms are uncontrolled. **Stepwise progression** of additional medications may be required. Follow the **guidance** of the British Thoracic Society–Scottish Intercollegiate Guidelines Network (BTS–SIGN) and the National Institute for Clinical Excellence (NICE) for diagnosis and treatment.

23 Assessing respiratory function

Figure 23.1 Peak flow meter

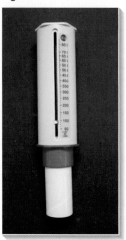

Figure 23.2 Spirometer

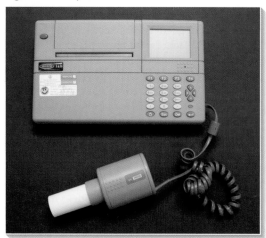

Figure 23.3 A trace from a spirometer

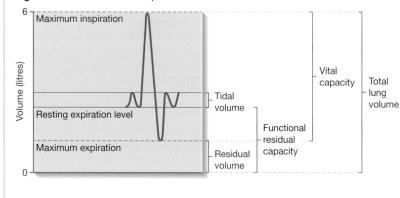

Figure 23.4 Flow volume loop

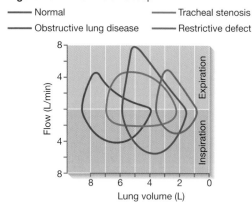

Table 23.1 Restrictive versus obstructive disorders

	FEV_1	FVC	FEV_1/FVC ratio	TLC	RV
Normal	↔	↔	>0.8	↔	↔
Obstructive	↓	↓ or ↔	<0.7	↓ or ↔	↑
Restrictive	↓	↓	>0.7	↓	↓

Box 23.1 Respiratory function test definitions

- **Forced vital capacity (FVC):** The amount of air from full inspiration to forced maximal expiration.
- **Forced expiratory volume in one second (FEV_1):** The amount of air forcefully exhaled during one second.
- **FEV_1–FVC ratio:** is the ratio of the forced expiratory volume in one second to the forced vital capacity of the lungs.
- **Tidal volume (TV):** The amount of air inhaled and exhaled during normal breathing at rest.
- **Total lung capacity (TLC):** The maximum volume of air present in the lungs.
- **Residual volume (RV):** The amount of air remaining in the lungs after maximum exhalation.

Practical Medical Procedures At a Glance, First Edition. Rachel K. Thomas © Rachel K. Thomas. Published 2015 by John Wiley & Sons, Ltd.
Companion website: http://www.ataglanceseries.com/practicalmedprocedures

What are respiratory function tests?

Respiratory function tests, including **peak flow** and **spirometry**, are simple tests performed to evaluate a patient's lungs function. A **peak expiratory flow meter** is a **small handheld device** that provides a simple way of **assessing upper airway status and monitoring response to medication**.

In **spirometry**, the patient breathes into a **spirometer**, which records various parameters such as the patient's **tidal volume**; **vital capacity**; **forced expiratory volume** (FEV_1), which is the volume expired in 1 second; and **forced vital capacity** (**FVC**) (Box 23.1). These are used to diagnose and monitor the progression of disease.

Why are respiratory function tests important?

Peak flow meters are **simple** to use and **inexpensive**, and they provide **convenient monitoring of the condition of the upper airways** and response to medication (Figure 23.1). They measure the maximum speed of exhalation in the FVC manoeuvre, and it is expressed in litres per minute. Values vary according to the patient's height, age and gender, and accurate readings depend on good technique. It is particularly useful for conditions such as asthma. Patients can easily monitor their normal peak flow readings to indicate illness severity – a typical pattern of dipping in the morning and improving throughout the day is common, whilst lower values are concerning: <50% of their normal value indicates a severe asthma attack, and <30% indicates a life-threatening attack.

Spirometry is a measure of flow and volume against time (Figure 23.2). It is used in the **diagnosis** and **monitoring** of conditions, such as asthma, chronic obstructive pulmonary disease (COPD) and pulmonary fibrosis; in **differentiating** between **restrictive** and **obstructive** disorders (Table 23.1); and in assessing the effects of **treatments**. Results are displayed as a **trace** (Figure 23.3) or as a **flow-volume loop** (Figure 23.4) giving more information on the **site** of airway narrowing.

Indications

- Respiratory disease such as asthma or COPD

Contra-indications

- Patient refusal

Complications

- **Local** – nil
- **Systemic** – fainting or syncope, inaccurate readings, diagnostic problems due to poor technique

Procedure

To measure peak flow:
- **Introduce** yourself, and **identify** the patient (see Chapter 4).
- Gain **consent** for the procedure (see Chapter 5), explain **indications** and check for **contra-indications** or **allergies**.
- Ensure **bare below the elbows**, and **wash hands** (see Chapter 6).
- Apply a **single-use disposable mouthpiece**.
- **Zero** the peak flow meter by sliding the indicator back towards the mouthpiece.
- Instruct patient to:
  - Stand or sit **upright**.
  - Take as **deep** a breath as possible.
  - Place the mouthpiece in his or her mouth, with the **tongue underneath** and lips **tightly closed** around the mouthpiece, and **blow out as hard and as fast as possible**.
  - Then breathe normally.
  - **Repeat** the process twice more (ideally, leaving 30 seconds between attempts).
- Record the best of **three readings**.
- Readings should be similar in value. Otherwise, check technique and repeat at an appropriate time, taking care not to exhaust the patient.
- **Thank patient**, and ensure that they are comfortable and have no adverse effects.
- **Dispose** of mouthpiece in clinical waste bin.
- **Wash hands**.

Did you know?

Total lung capacity cannot be estimated from spirometry. It is measured using **inspiration** of a **gas** (e.g. helium) and recording the **dilution** of this gas with the gas in the lungs, or by a technique called **plethysmography**.

To perform spirometry:
- **Introduce** yourself, and **identify** the patient (see Chapter 4).
- Gain **consent** for the procedure (see Chapter 5), explain **indications** and check for **contra-indications**.
- Ensure **bare below the elbows**, and **wash hands** (see Chapter 6).
- Get the patient **sitting comfortably**, and allow them to have some **practice attempts**. **Demonstrate the technique**. **Take care not to exhaust the patient**.
- Record the patient's **age**, **sex** and **height**.
- Apply a **nose clip**.
- Attach a **single-use mouthpiece** to the device and place in the patient's mouth, ensuring that the lips are sealed around the device with the tongue underneath.
- For FEV_1 or **FVC**:
  - Ask the patient to breathe in as deeply as possible, and then breathe out as hard and as fast as possible until there is nothing left to expel. Encourage actively.
  - Repeat this twice until at least two values are within 5% or 100 ml of each other.
- For **vital capacity**:
  - Record while the patient is breathing out at a comfortable pace.
- Record the readings.
- **Thank patient**, and ensure that they are comfortable and have no adverse effects.
- Dispose of mouthpiece in clinical waste bin.
- **Wash hands**.

24 Using airway manoeuvres and simple adjuncts

Figure 24.1 Airway care and adjuncts *in situ*. Source: Blundell and Harrison (2013), Chapter 13, Station 30 p. 38.

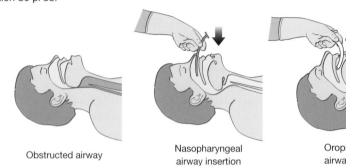
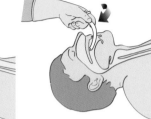
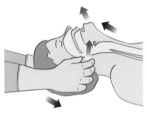
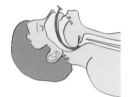
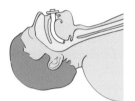

Obstructed airway

Nasopharyngeal airway insertion

Oropharyngeal airway insertion

Head tilt, chin lift, jaw thrust

Nasopharyngeal airway in situ

Oropharyngeal airway in situ

Figure 24.2 Naso-pharyngeal airways – older designs need an additional pin to increase the flange diameter

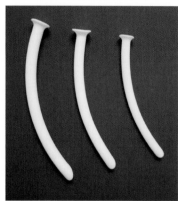

(a)

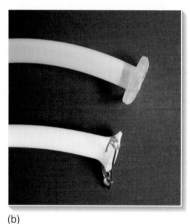

(b)

Figure 24.3 Oropharangeal airways

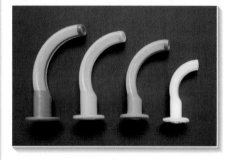

Figure 24.4 Laryngeal mask airway

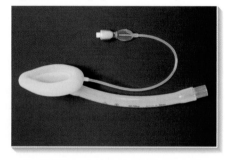

Figure 24.5 I-gel® airway

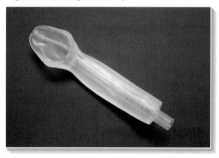

Figure 24.6 Endotracheal tube

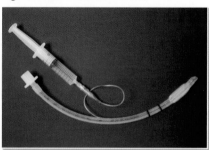

Hints and tips:

- **Head tilt** and **chin lift** should be avoided in patients with a suspected **cervical spine injury – jaw thrust** is preferred.
- Only use **suction** under **direct vision**.
- **Reassess the effect** of each intervention.
- **Ensure you inform a senior** of the patient's condition.

What are airway manoeuvres and simple adjuncts?

Airway manoeuvres are **three simple manoeuvres** that can be used to open an obstructed or partially obstructed airway (Figure 24.1). These are:

- **Head tilt**
- **Chin lift**
- **Jaw thrust**.

Head tilt and **chin lift** are carried out together by placing one hand on the patient's forehead and applying gentle downward pressure to **tilt** the head back, whilst the other hand is placed under the chin and **lifted**. A **jaw thrust** brings the **lower jaw** (mandible) **forwards** and **upwards**. Place your four fingers behind the angle of the mandible, and apply upwards and forwards pressure in order to **relieve obstruction** by the tongue and epiglottis. Open the patient's mouth by moving the **chin downwards** with your thumbs.

Airway adjuncts are pieces of **equipment** that help to **maintain an open airway**, and they may need to be used in conjunction with **simple manoeuvres** (Figure 24.1). The main types of airway adjuncts you may need to use are:

- **Nasopharyngeal airway** (Figure 24.2a and Figure 24.2b)
- **Oropharyngeal airway** (or Guedel airway) (Figure 24.3).

A **nasopharyngeal airway** (Figure 24.2), a **small tube** passed via the **nostril**, is **tolerated** better than an oropharyngeal airway and can be used in patients with an **intact gag reflex**. It should not be used in someone with a skull base fracture unless the benefits outweigh the risks. Usually, a **size 6–7** is suitable for an adult.

The **oropharyngeal airway** or **Guedel airway** (Figure 24.3) is a curved plastic tube which is inserted into the airway through the **mouth** to maintain an open airway in an **unconscious** patient. It is **not tolerated** in patients with an **intact gag reflex**. Simple manoeuvres may still be required to maintain an open airway. To size, measure from the **incisor** to the **angle of the jaw**.

Other adjuncts, such as the **laryngeal mask airway (LMA)** (Figure 24.4), **I-gels** (Figure 24.5) and **endotracheal tube (ET)** (Figure 24.6), are beyond the scope of this book. These adjuncts are for use only in unconscious patients. **LMAs** and **I-gels** are both **supraglottic airways**, where a mask sits above the vocal cords. An **ET** passes through the vocal cords into the trachea, and it is a **definitive airway** which is inserted under general anaesthetic by trained experts only.

Why are airway manoeuvres and adjuncts important?

These manoeuvers and airway adjuncts are important in the treatment of an **obstructed** or **partially obstructed airway**. To assess for airway obstruction, **look** for chest and abdominal movement, **listen** for airflow at the mouth and nose and **feel** for airflow at the mouth and nose.

Signs of **partial airway obstruction** may include wheeze (lower airway obstruction), stridor (upper airway obstruction), gurgling (liquid) and snoring (occlusion of pharynx by the tongue).

In **complete airway obstruction**, there is seesaw breathing (paradoxical respiration), where the patient's chest is drawn in and their abdomen expands with inspiration – the opposite of normal.

The patient may also be using **accessory muscles** in order to breathe.

Indications
- Obstructed or partially obstructed airway
- Aiding ventilation

Contra-indications
- Base-of-skull fracture if nasopharyngeal adjunct
- Patient refusal

Complications
- **Local** – trigger gag reflex if reflex intact, bleeding, trauma
- **Systemic** – hypoxaemia if incorrectly inserted

Procedure

For nasopharyngeal airway adjunct insertion:

- Check whether the right nostril is **patent (preferred unless blocked)**.
- Insert **safety pin** through flange of adjunct if required (Figure 24.2b).
- **Lubricate** the adjunct with **water-based lubricant**.
- Insert the airway along the **floor of the nose**, advancing gently in a posterior direction. Avoid force, especially in a superior direction.
- Check airway **patency** using look, listen and feel.
- **Airway manoeuvres may still be required**.

For oropharyngeal airway adjunct insertion:

- **Measure** from incisor to angle of the jaw.
- Open the patient's mouth, and ensure that nothing is obstructing the airway.
- If an obstruction is **seen**, use **suction** to extract it.
- Insert the airway adjunct **upside down**, with the hollow end of the tube pointing upwards towards the hard palate to avoid the tongue. A tongue depressor may be used.
- **Rotate** it 180° once you reach the soft palate; perform this step gently, avoiding trauma.
- Advance until the flattened end of the airway is between the patient's teeth.
- **Airway manoeuvres may still be required**.

25 Ventilating with a bag valve mask device

Figure 25.1 Equipment required for ventilation

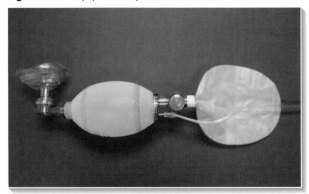

Figure 25.2 Two-handed technique

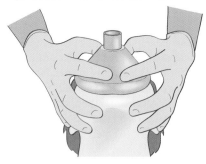

Figure 25.3 Bag valve mask

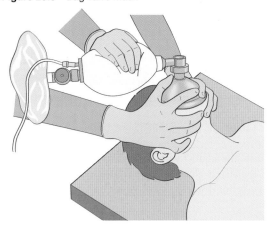

Figure 25.4 Suction device

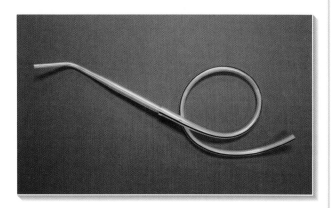

Figure 25.5 Masks come in different sizes

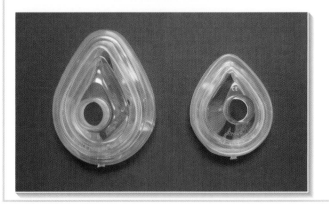

Hints and tips:

- If there is a problem with ventilation, check the **seal** of the mask, the patient's **position**, your **hold** on the mask and your use of **airway adjuncts**.
- Use the **two person** technique for ventilation.
- Look for signs of **reversible causes** of **hypoventilation**, such as an **opiate overdose** – check for **pinpoint pupils** and consider treatment with **naloxone** (given by IV injection, 0.4–2 mg, repeated every 2–3 min to a maximum of 10 mg).
- Ultimately **endotracheal intubation** is the best way of ventilating an unconscious patient – for **maintenance** and **protection** of the airway!
- Call for help earlier rather than later.

Practical Medical Procedures at a Glance, First Edition. Rachel K. Thomas © Rachel K. Thomas. Published 2015 by John Wiley & Sons, Ltd.
Companion website: http://www.ataglanceseries.com/practicalmedprocedures

What is a bag valve mask device?

A **bag valve mask device** is an **airway device** that consists of a **self-inflating bag** attached to a **one-way valve** which attaches to a **face mask**, tracheal tube or supraglottic device (Figure 25.1). When the bag is squeezed, its contents (oxygen or air) are delivered directly to the patient. The purpose is to inflate the lungs. Expired gas is expelled into the atmosphere via the valve.

A bag valve mask can be used in conjunction with **airway adjuncts** such as oropharyngeal or nasopharyngeal airways (see Chapter 24). It is preferable to have at least **two people** present to use the bag valve mask: one person performs basic airway manoeuvres whilst maintaining a seal with the face mask, using two hands and standing behind the patient's head (Figure 25.2). The second person squeezes the bag to inflate the lungs (Figure 25.3).

A complete absence of respiratory or cardiac effort requires commencement of cardiopulmonary resuscitation immediately and help – such as the arrest team (see Chapter 27).

Why is a bag valve mask device important?

This device enables oxygen or air to be delivered to a patient who is **not breathing** (apnoeic) or who is **breathing too infrequently** (hypoventilation). It should be present on all **resuscitation trolleys**. In an emergency setting, the bag should always be connected to an **oxygen** supply rather than air. It is used during arrest or peri-arrest situations and anaesthesia.

A **wide-bore suction device** (called a 'Yankauer') can be used to **remove secretions** from the upper airway (Figure 25.4). This may induce gagging or vomiting, and should always be done under direct vision.

Indications

- Hypoventilation
- Peri-arrest, arrest emergency situations

Contra-indications

- In some circumstances – a clearly and correctly documented 'Do Not Attempt Resuscitation' order

Complications

- **Local** – trauma
- **Systemic** – inflation of the stomach

Procedure

Holding the mask:

- Select the appropriate size, based on the size of the patient's face, so that it covers the nose and mouth (Figure 25.5).
- Ensure **bare below the elbows**, and **wash hands** (see Chapter 6).
- Don personal protective equipment as required.
- Hold the mask so that your thumb and index finger make a **C-shape** around the mask on each side. The remaining three fingers should be positioned **under the patient's jaw** so as to tilt the patient's head and elevate the jaw to open the airway (Figure 25.2).

Performing the bag valve mask ventilation:

- Assess airway patency.
- Suction secretions if required.
- Perform **head tilt**, **chin lift** and **jaw thrust**.
- Site **oropharyngeal** or **nasopharyngeal airway** as tolerated, if needed (see Chapter 24).
- Attach **oxygen** if available.
- Begin resuscitation via bag valve mask. A**im for 10 to 12 breaths per minute (this requires squeezing the bag once every 5 to 6 seconds). The bag should be depressed for approximately one second, and then released.**
- **Summon help as soon as possible.**

Did you know?

To assess ventilation clinically:
- **Look** to see if the **chest** is rising and falling.
- **Look** for condensation on the **mask**.
- **Listen** to the **chest** for breath sounds.

The best way to assess if ventilation is adequate is by **capnography**, which measures **end tidal carbon dioxide levels**. This should produce a **trace** that **rises** and **falls** with each breath.

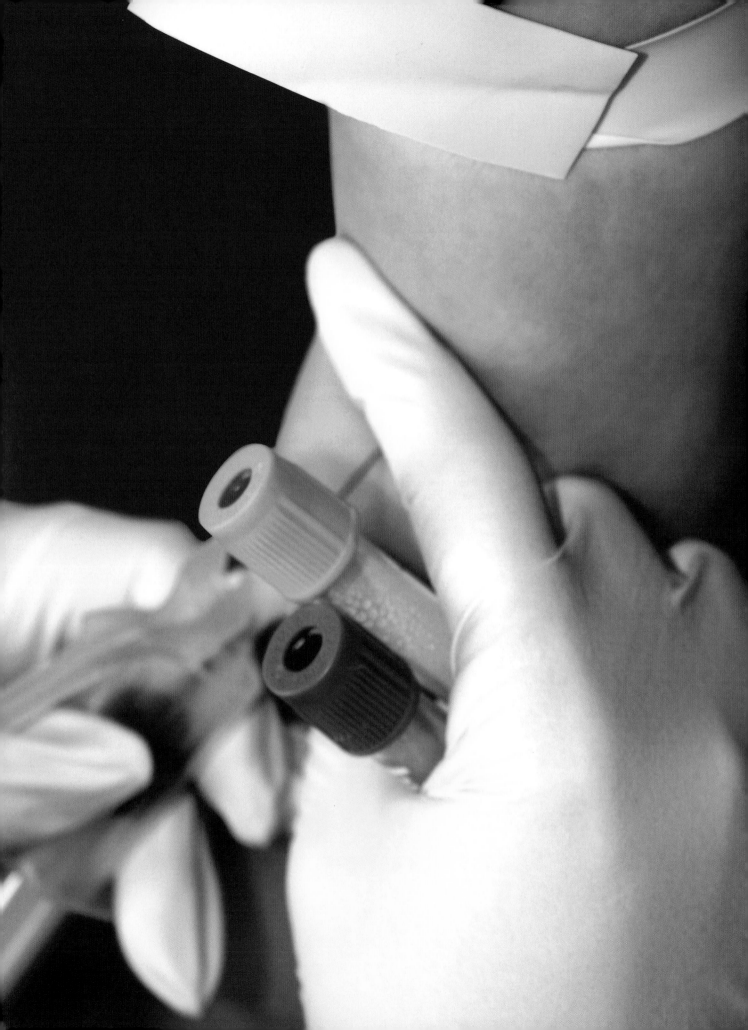

Common procedures – cardiology

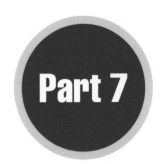

Part 7

Chapters

26 Recording a 12-lead electrocardiogram 64
27 Performing cardiopulmonary resuscitation 66

26 Recording a 12-lead electrocardiogram

Figure 26.1 Electrode positions for chest leads for electrocardiogram (ECG)

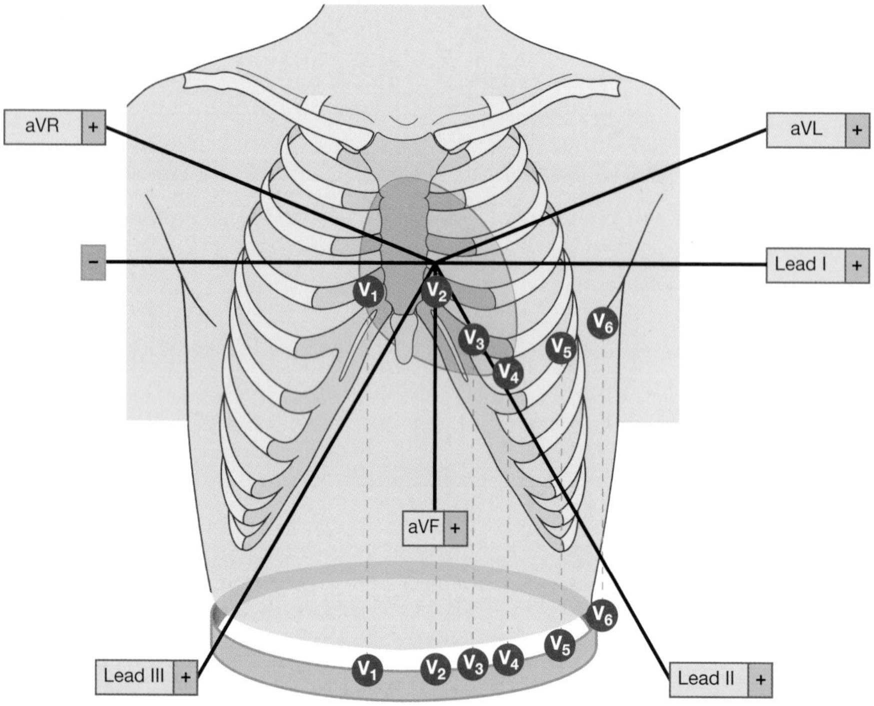

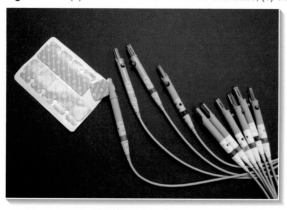

aVR +

aVL +

−

Lead I +

V₁ V₂ V₃ V₄ V₅ V₆

aVF +

Lead III +

Lead II +

Figure 26.2 (a) Electrode adhesive stickers and leads; (b) electrode attached to the wrist

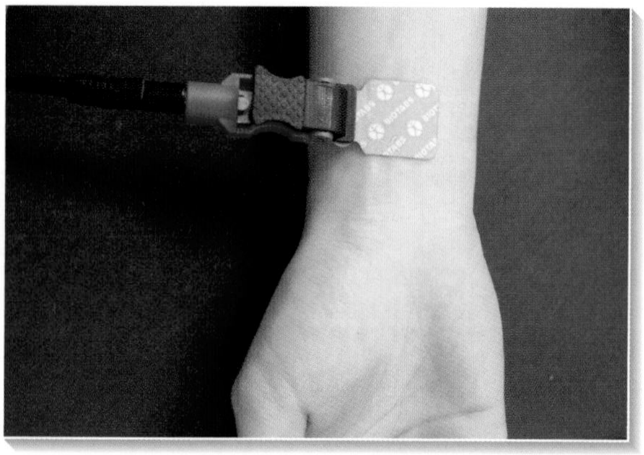

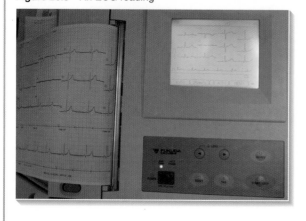

Figure 26.3 An ECG reading

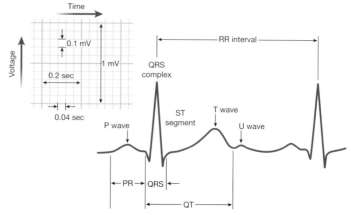

Figure 26.4 The main waves and intervals

Time

Voltage

0.1 mV

1 mV

0.2 sec

0.04 sec

RR interval

QRS complex

ST segment

T wave

U wave

P wave

PR → QRS ←

QT

Practical Medical Procedures at a Glance, First Edition. Rachel K. Thomas © Rachel K. Thomas. Published 2015 by John Wiley & Sons, Ltd.
Companion website: http://www.ataglanceseries.com/practicalmedprocedures

What is an electrocardiogram?

An **electrocardiogram (ECG)** is a tracing of the **electrical activity** of the heart. It is performed using **10 electrode pads** that are placed on the patient's limbs (**four** electrodes) and chest (**six** electrodes) (Figure 26.1). Wires from an **ECG machine** are attached to the electrodes (Figure 26.2). Wires V1, V2, V3, V4, V5 and V6 connect to the chest electrodes, whilst wires RA (right arm; red colour), LA (left arm; yellow), LL (left leg; green) and RL (right leg; blue or black) connect to the limb electrodes (Figure 26.2a and 26.2b). With the patient lying **still**, the machine detects the **electrical activity** from the **heart muscle** and produces a reading.

Although there are only 10 electrodes, the ECG machine produces a reading of the heart from **12 views**, also referred to as 'leads' (Figure 26.3). Thus, it is often referred to as a **12-lead ECG**, with each lead 'looking' at a different view of the heart. The different leads look at different views of the heart – Leads V1–V4 look at the **anterior aspect** of the heart (with V1 and V2 looking at the **septum**). Leads I, aVL, V5 and V6 look at the **lateral aspect**, while Leads aVF, II and III look at the **inferior aspect** (Figure 26.1).

Similarly, **cardiac monitoring** can be performed using **three** electrodes and three wires – the **red**, **yellow** and **green** – to produce a **continuous tracing** (which is part of the standard 12-lead ECG, **lead II**, commonly referred to as the 'rhythm strip'). For cardiac monitoring, place the electrode pads over the **right** and **left shoulders**, and the **apex beat**, respectively, and connect the specified three wires appropriately.

The **positive deflection** in an ECG waveform represents when the **depolarisation** of that region of muscle is **flowing towards** the electrode.

Why is an electrocardiogram important?

An ECG gives us vital information about the **heart's activity**, **disease** processes affecting the heart and the patient's **overall health**.

It can be interpreted by looking at various components (Figure 26.4). These include:
- **Heart rate**. Is the patient **tachycardic** (heart rate >100) or **bradycardic** (heart rate <60)?
- **Rhythm**. Is it regular sinus rhythm, or is it an irregular rhythm such as atrial fibrillation?
- **Axis**. What is the overall direction of the flow of electrical activity?
- Are there **P** waves present – suggestive of atrial depolarisation?
- What is the **PR interval**?
- Are the **QRS complexes** narrow or broad?
- Are the **T waves** normal? Or inverted? Or tented?

This is only a brief list – a thorough understanding of the interpretation of ECGs is necessary for every doctor and not covered here.

Indications
- Clinical suspicion of cardiac pathology, chest pain, shortness of breath
- Monitoring – of medications, in theatre
- Metabolic derangement

Contra-indications
- Patient refusal

Complications
- **Local** – skin reaction
- **Systemic** – nil

Procedure

- **Introduce** yourself, and **identify** the patient (see Chapter 4).
- Gain **consent** for the procedure (see Chapter 5), explain **indications** and check for **contra-indications** or **allergies** or previous reactions to the electrode adhesive.
- Ensure **bare below the elbows**, and **wash hands** (see Chapter 6).
- Collect the **ECG machine** and the **adhesive electrode pads**.
- Offer a **chaperone**.
- Position the patient **sitting back** and comfortable with their chest exposed; ensure that skin is **clean** and **dry**.
- If a patient is very **hairy**, it may be necessary to **shave** their skin to enable good electrode contact.
- Check the ECG machine, power cable, patient lead cables and paper, and attach machine to power socket.
- Turn ECG machine on, start self-test analysis and **check machine calibration**.
- To obtain a 12-lead ECG, place the **adhesive electrode pads** in the correct locations (named according to the wire which will connect to it) on the **chest** and the **limbs**:
  - **Chest** – find the fourth intercostal space, on either side of the sternum, and the fifth intercostal space in the mid-clavicular and mid-axillary lines (**hint**: The second intercostal space is reliably identified by palpation of the manubriosternal joint as the second pair of ribs attach here):
    - **V1** – right fourth intercostal space, next to sternum
    - **V2** – left fourth intercostal space, next to sternum
    - **V4** – left fifth intercostal space, mid-clavicular line
    - **V6** – left fifth intercostal space, mid-axillary line
    - **V3** – place evenly between **V2** and **V4**
    - **V5** – anterior axillary line is level with **V4**.
  - **Limb** – place on the **outer aspect of each forearm** and the **medial aspect of each lower leg** (or on each shoulder and hip, ensuring consistency for comparison of readings):
    - **Red (RA)**: right arm
    - **Yellow (LA)**: left arm
    - **Green (LL)**: left leg
    - **Black (RL)**: right leg
- **Attach** the electrode wires onto the **adhesive electrode pads** – six on the chest and the four on the limbs.
- Ask the patient to **breathe normally** and **remain still**, while a tracing is obtained and printed out.
- Record on the ECG reading the patient's details, the time, the date and any **symptoms** the patient was having at the time of the ECG.
- Before disconnection, double check to ensure that the recording:
  - Is free from artefacts such as movement
  - Reflects correct lead placement
  - Shows correct calibration for paper speed of 25 mm/s
  - Shows correct calibration for voltage of 1 mV/10 mm.
- **Turn off** ECG machine.
- **Disconnect wires** from **adhesive electrode pads**, and remove any gel or residue remaining on the patient.
- Dispose of waste in clinical waste bins.
- **Wash hands**.
- **Thank patient**, and ensure that they are comfortable and have no adverse effects.
- Interpret the ECG reading, seeking senior input for interpretation if required.

Did you know?

The paper needs to run at the **standard rate** of **25 mm/s**, and the **voltage** calibrated to **1 mV** represents **10 mm** vertically. Most doctors can recall a time when a patient's ECG showed severe abnormalities, yet clinically they were asymptomatic – because it was due to the paper running through at the wrong speed!

Performing cardiopulmonary resuscitation

Figure 27.1 Cardiopulmonary resuscitation and defibrillation. Adapted from Blundell and Harrison (2013) Chapter 13, p. 38, and Carney and Gallen (2014), Figure 19.1, p. 52.

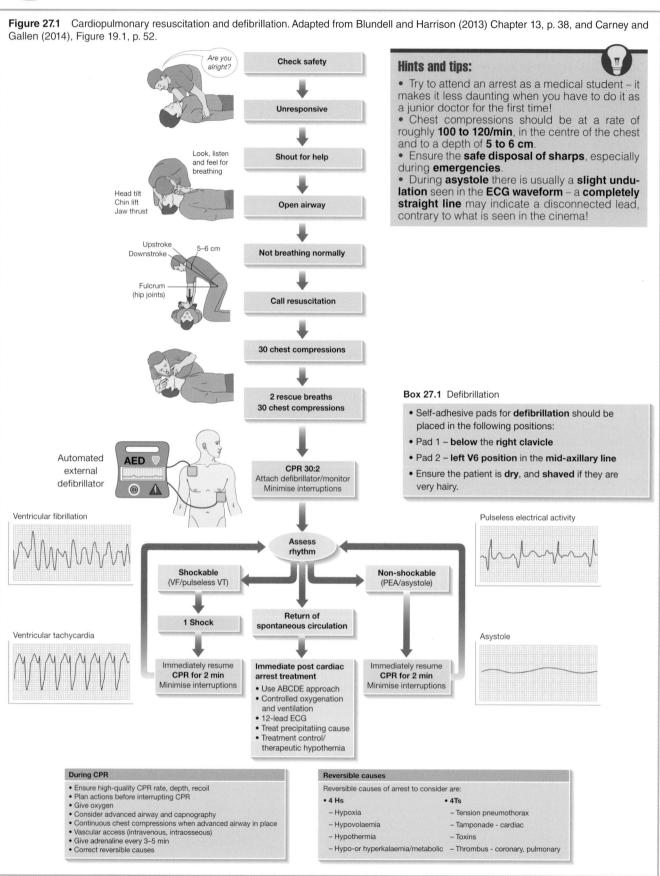

Hints and tips:

- Try to attend an arrest as a medical student – it makes it less daunting when you have to do it as a junior doctor for the first time!
- Chest compressions should be at a rate of roughly **100 to 120/min**, in the centre of the chest and to a depth of **5 to 6 cm**.
- Ensure the **safe disposal of sharps**, especially during **emergencies**.
- During **asystole** there is usually a **slight undulation** seen in the **ECG waveform** – a **completely straight line** may indicate a disconnected lead, contrary to what is seen in the cinema!

Box 27.1 Defibrillation

- Self-adhesive pads for **defibrillation** should be placed in the following positions:
- Pad 1 – **below** the **right clavicle**
- Pad 2 – **left V6 position** in the **mid-axillary line**
- Ensure the patient is **dry**, and **shaved** if they are very hairy.

During CPR

- Ensure high-quality CPR rate, depth, recoil
- Plan actions before interrupting CPR
- Give oxygen
- Consider advanced airway and capnography
- Continuous chest compressions when advanced airway in place
- Vascular access (intravenous, intraosseous)
- Give adrenaline every 3–5 min
- Correct reversible causes

Reversible causes

Reversible causes of arrest to consider are:

• 4 Hs	• 4Ts
– Hypoxia	– Tension pneumothorax
– Hypovolaemia	– Tamponade - cardiac
– Hypothermia	– Toxins
– Hypo-or hyperkalaemia/metabolic	– Thrombus - coronary, pulmonary

Practical Medical Procedures at a Glance, First Edition. Rachel K. Thomas © Rachel K. Thomas. Published 2015 by John Wiley & Sons, Ltd.
Companion website: http://www.ataglanceseries.com/practicalmedprocedures

What is cardiopulmonary resuscitation?

Cardiopulmonary resuscitation (CPR) is the technique used to maintain a person's cardiac and respiratory output when they are in cardiac and/or respiratory arrest. There are **standardised algorithms** for CPR which must be adhered to, which are available from resources such as the Resuscitation Council.

Why is cardiopulmonary resuscitation important?

CPR is important in an **emergency** to maintain **perfusion** of vital organs until further action can be taken, such as treating **reversible causes** and/or **defibrillation** (Figure 27.1). A **defibrillator** is a device that shows the **rhythm** of the heart, and then can be used to deliver an **electric shock** to the heart in an attempt to revert it to a normal sinus rhythm and restore cardiac output. **Self-adhesive pads** from the defibrillator are attached to the **chest** in specific locations (Box 27.1). Whether or not defibrillation is required during CPR depends on the type of rhythm seen during the arrest. **Ventricular tachycardia (VT)** and **ventricular fibrillation (VF)** are considered **shockable** and thus require defibrillation. **Asystole** and **pulseless electrical activity (PEA)** are **non-shockable** rhythms, and thus are not defibrillated.

Indications
- Unresponsive patient

Contra-indications
- Clearly and correctly documented 'Do Not Attempt Resuscitation' order

Complications
- **Local** – pain, fractures, bruising
- **Systemic** – organ damage from poor perfusion

Procedure

For an unresponsive patient:
- Assess for danger.
- Is the patient responsive?
- Shout for help.
- **Airway**: head tilt, chin lift, jaw thrust.
- **Breathing** and circulation: look, listen and feel for 10 seconds for signs of life. May feel for a carotid pulse.
- If no evidence of breathing or circulation, call the **cardiac arrest team**.
- Start chest **compressions** at a rate of **30 compressions to 2 breaths** (30:2) until intubated.

- Apply **self-adhesive defibrillation pads once help arrives**.
- Stop chest compressions only **momentarily** to confirm rhythm on ECG.

If the ECG shows a shockable rhythm:
- *Restart chest compressions without delay, as the designated person selects the correct energy on the defibrillator and charges it.
- All rescuers should stand clear except the person performing chest compressions.
- As soon as the defibrillator has finished charging, advise the person performing chest compressions to step away.
- **Give the shock.**
- **Restart CPR immediately.**
- **Continue for 2 minutes.**
- Pause CPR to check monitor, **minimising the pause**.
- If it is a shockable rhythm, repeat from* (first item of this sublist), and deliver a second shock.
- If VF or VT is still present, repeat from* and shock the patient for a third time. Immediately restart chest compressions, and then give **1 mg intravenous (IV) adrenaline** and **300 mg IV amiodarone** whilst continuing CPR.
- Repeat the 2-minute cycle if VF or VT persists.
- Give further **adrenaline** after **alternate shocks**.

If the ECG shows a non-shockable rhythm:
- Start **CPR 30:2**.
- Give **adrenaline 1 mg IV** as soon as IV access is achieved.
- Continue CPR 30:2 until the airway is secured.
- **Recheck** the rhythm after 2 minutes:
  - If you observe **organised electrical activity**, then look for signs of life and check for a pulse.
    If these are present, begin post-resuscitation care.
    If these are not present, continue CPR, and do not check the rhythm until 2 minutes have passed. **Every 3–5 minutes**, give further **adrenaline 1 mg IV** (during alternate loops of CPR).
  - If you observe VF or VT, swap to the shockable algorithm.
  - If you observe asystole or agonal rhythms, continue CPR, and do not check the rhythm until 2 minutes have passed. **Every 3–5 minutes**, give further **adrenaline 1 mg IV** (during alternate loops of CPR).

Did you know?
For shockable rhythms:
   Adrenaline is given at a dose of **1 mg IV** after the **third shock**, and then after **alternate shocks**.
   Amiodarone is given for **shockable** rhythms only, at a dose of 300 mg IV after the **third shock**.
For non-shockable rhythms:
   Adrenaline is given at a dose of **1 mg IV**, given **immediately** when venous access is achieved and then every **3–5 minutes**.

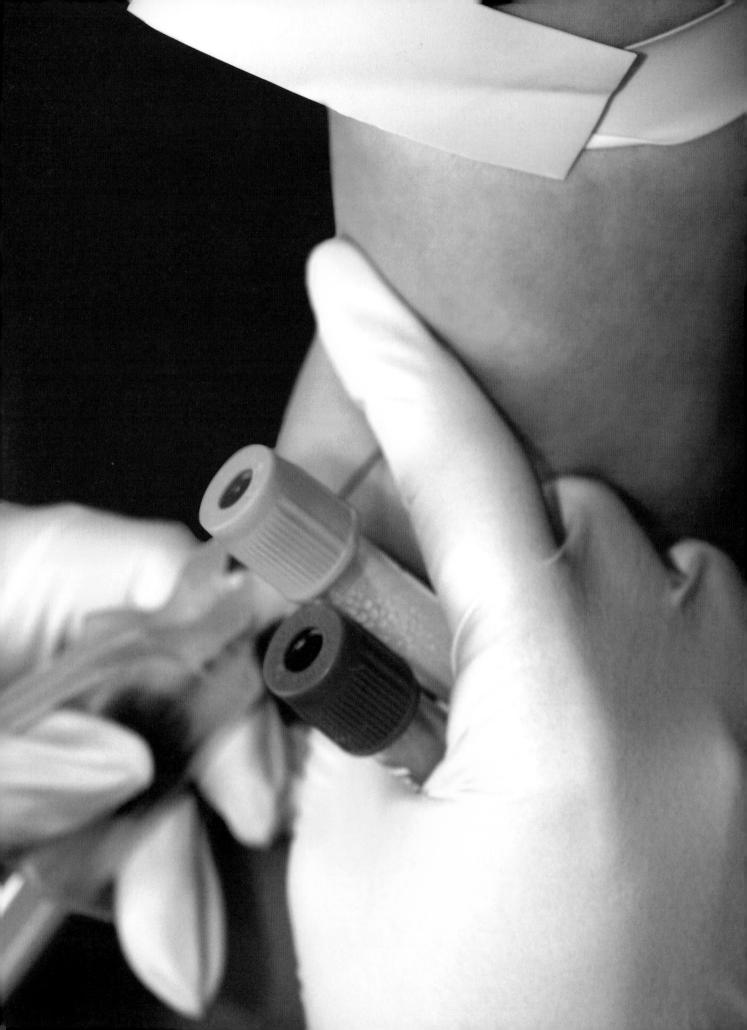

Common procedures – gastroenterology

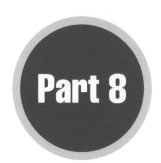

Part 8

Chapters

28   **Inserting a nasogastric tube**   70

29   **Performing a digital rectal examination**   72

28 Inserting a nasogastric tube

Figure 28.1   Route of nasogastric tube and sizing landmarks

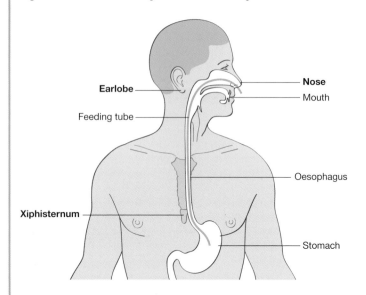

Nose
Mouth
Earlobe
Feeding tube
Oesophagus
Xiphisternum
Stomach

Figure 28.2   Patient position for insertion

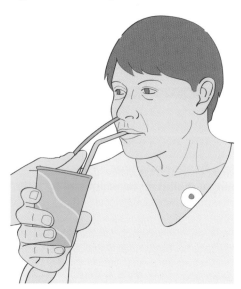

Figure 28.3   (a) A fine-bore nasogastric tube, and (b) a large bore (Ryle's) tube with drainage bag attached

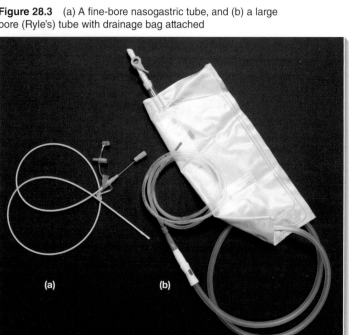

(a)   (b)

Figure 28.4   Chest X-ray showing correctly sited nosogastric tube. Source: Blundell and Harrison (2013), Chapter 28, p. 70.

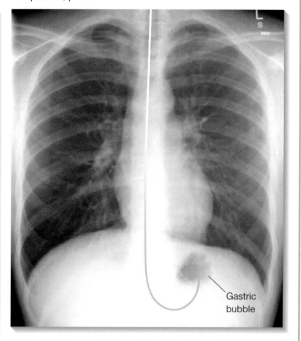

Gastric bubble

What is a nasogastric tube?

A **nasogastric (NG) tube** is a **narrow plastic tube** that is inserted into the stomach via the nostril. These tubes are of different **bores**, or diameters, depending on their clinical indication. It is important to ensure that the correct length of tube is inserted. To measure the required length of tube, measure from the tip of the **patient's nose**, to their **ear**, and then down to the **xiphisternum** (Figure 28.1). A typical length would be approximately 50–60 cm, which can be noted and halted at when the tube is introduced (Figure 28.2).

Why is a nasogastric tube important?

Nasogastric tubes can be inserted for a variety of reasons – the main indications are either to **introduce substances** into, or to **remove substances** from, the stomach. There are two main types of nasogastric tube. A **large-bore** (or Ryle's) tube (Figure 28.3b) is used for stomach decompression and removal of its contents, as in bowel obstruction – a **drainage bag** is fixed to the end of the tube. A **fine-bore** tube (Figure 28.3a) is used for enteral feeding – an **enteral nutrition bag** is fixed to the end of the tube.

Practical Medical Procedures at a Glance, First Edition. Rachel K. Thomas © Rachel K. Thomas. Published 2015 by John Wiley & Sons, Ltd.
Companion website: http://www.ataglanceseries.com/practicalmedprocedures

Always ensure the nasogastric tube is **correctly sited** prior to use for feeding. Ensure that you adhere to local policies – most local policies require a senior physician to **verify correct tube placement prior to use** for feeding, and the gold standard for confirming the site is on a **chest X-ray** (Figure 28.4). The tip of the NG tube should be seen in the gastric bubble, under the line of the diaphragm.

A careful **history** and **examination** of the patient are essential before insertion. Head and facial **trauma**, particularly **basal skull fracture** (sub-orbital bruising, or 'Panda eyes', and retro-auricular bruising, or 'Battel's sign'), are contra-indications to NG tube insertion.

Indications
- Stomach decompression
- Enteral feeding

Contra-indications
- Patient refusal
- Basal skull fracture

Complications
- **Local** – misplaced NG tube, tracheal insertion, pain, trauma
- **Systemic** – aspiration, infection, electrolyte imbalance

---

Procedure
- **Introduce** yourself, and **identify** the patient (see Chapter 4).
- Gain **consent** for the procedure (see Chapter 5), explain **indications** and check for **contra-indications** or **allergies**.
- Ensure **bare below the elbows, wash hands** and **don apron** (see Chapter 6).
- Wipe clean a **tray** with antibacterial wipes.
- Select the **appropriate bore tube** as clinically indicated.
- Collect equipment and place in the tray, including:
  - Non-sterile gloves and apron
  - Nasogastric tube
  - Lubricant or container of water
  - Specialised dressing or fixative tape
  - Cup of water for the patient.
- **Wash hands**, and put on **non-sterile gloves.**
- **Position** the patient so that they are **sitting upright** with their head slightly forwards (Figure 28.2).
- **Examine nostrils** and **nasal passages** to ensure that they are suitable for insertion.
- **Measure** tube length required, from the patient's **nostril** to their **ear** to their **xiphisternum**, and record length (Figure 28.1).
- Warn them of an **initial discomfort** – lidocaine spray can be sprayed in the nostril if the patient is concerned about pain on insertion.
- Ask the patient to take a **sip** of water and hold it in their mouth.
- Apply **lubricant** to the tube (water for a fine-bore feeding tube, and KY jelly for a large-bore tube).
- Insert the tube into the nostril, aiming directly **back** (not up, as may seem instinctively appropriate).
- Ask the patient to **swallow** the water once they feel the tube at the back of their throat.

- Continue passing the tube into the patient until the **pre-measured length** is reached.
- Remove the guide wire if present, or attach to a drainage bag if required.
- Secure the tube with specialised dressing or fixative tape.
- **Document** in the patient's notes date, time, signature, designation and any difficulties encountered.
- **Aspirate** the contents present at the end of the tube and place on a pH strip, and check acidity to help indicate stomach placement.
- Dispose of waste in clinical waste bins, and clean the tray.
- **Wash hands**.
- **Order a chest X-ray, document that this has been ordered, and await confirmation of the correct position before the tube is used for feeding**.
- **Thank patient**, and ensure that they are comfortable and have no adverse effects.

Hints and tips:
- Always **verify correct tube placement prior to use** – if incorrectly placed, and used for feeding, aspiration pneumonia and death may occur.
- Stomach juices are very **acidic** (pH <3). If the pH is higher than 5, it may be in the wrong place.
- **'Spigotting'** the tube means clamping or capping the end of it, so that it is not open or draining.
- If you are unsure if a patient needs an NG tube, discuss with your **seniors**, the **Speech and Language Therapy (SALT)** team and **dietitians**.

Aspects of feeding

When they are unwell, patients may have **higher energy requirements** than when they are in good health, due to disease processes. This is often compounded by a **decreased appetite** and **decreased oral intake**.

A **nutritional assessment** should also be made of patients. This should be evaluated not only in patients requiring feeding via an NG tube, but in **all** patients in hospital. This includes assessment of their **general condition**, their **diet** and their **Body Mass Index (BMI)**. Their **height** and **weight** must be measured and recorded, in order to calculate their BMI (weight (kg) / height (m²)). This helps determine if they are underweight (<18.5), normal weight (18.5–25), overweight (25–29.9) or obese (30–39.9).

Specific deficiencies, such as folate, thiamine and iron, should be treated appropriately. **Nutritional support**, if required, may be provided via several **different routes**. It may be appropriate to encourage an increase in their **oral intake**, or to **prescribe fortified liquids** or **supplements**. In cases where an **NG tube** is inappropriate for feeding, other methods which are beyond the scope of this book may be used – methods such as a **percutaneous endoscopic gastrostomy (PEG)**, where a tube is surgically inserted into the stomach through the skin, and **total parenteral nutrition** (TPN), where nutrition is administered directly into the patient's vein.

Dietitians are usually available for additional **assistance** with assessing the nutritional status and nutritional requirements of patients, and for advice on nutritional support.

29 Performing a digital rectal examination

Figure 29.1 Relevant male anatomy

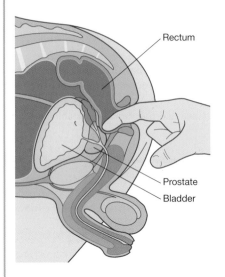

- Rectum
- Prostate
- Bladder

Figure 29.2 Relevant female anatomy

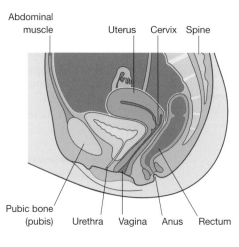

Abdominal muscle
Uterus Cervix Spine
Pubic bone (pubis) Urethra Vagina Anus Rectum

Figure 29.3 Lateral position for examination

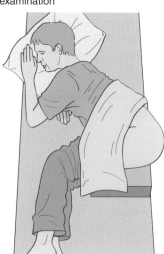

Figure 29.4 Performing a digital rectal examination

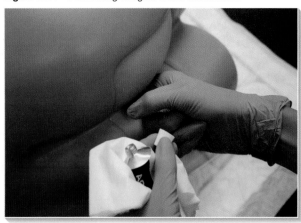

Did you know?

After performing a digital rectal examination, you must document your findings in the notes.
- Important findings include the following:
- Date, time, your designation
- Was a **chaperone** present?
- Did you see anything on **inspection** of the anus?
- Was **anal tone** normal? Was there normal sensation around the anus?
- Did you **palpate** anything? For example, was there hard faeces in the rectum? Was there a mass?
- (In males:) Did you feel the **prostate**? Was it enlarged? Did it feel smooth or irregular? Was it firm or hard? Did you feel a central sulcus?
- Was there blood on your finger when you removed it?

Hints and tips:

- Maintain the patient's **dignity** by performing the examination in a **private** room or with the curtains firmly closed.
- Warn the patient of the **cool lubricant** on the **gloved finger** prior to its insertion.
- Reassure the patient that the procedure may be **uncomfortable**, but should not hurt.

Practical Medical Procedures at a Glance, First Edition. Rachel K. Thomas © Rachel K. Thomas. Published 2015 by John Wiley & Sons, Ltd.
Companion website: http://www.ataglanceseries.com/practicalmedprocedures

What is a digital rectal exam?

A **digital rectal exam (DRE)** is the insertion of a gloved, lubricated finger into the **back passage** to examine for abnormalities. It is often referred to colloquially as a PR – short for *per rectum*.

Why are digital rectal examinations important?

A digital rectal examination is a quick, harmless and effective method of examining the anus, rectum and prostate gland in males (Figure 29.1). It is also useful in examining the female pelvis (Figure 29.2).

These simple examinations can help diagnose pathologies such as rectal or prostate cancer, and they are important in the investigation of many conditions from constipation to spinal cord compression.

Indications

- Diagnosis of prostate or rectal cancers
- Investigating bleeding from the back passage, or bowel habit change
- Part of neurological, abdominal and gynaecological examinations

Contra-indications

- Patient refusal
- Children (except in very specific circumstances)

Complications

- **Local** – discomfort
- **Systemic** – emotional discomfort

Procedure

- **Introduce** yourself, and **identify** the patient (see Chapter 4).
- Ask if the patient would like a **chaperone**.
- Gain **consent** for the procedure (see Chapter 5), explain **indications** and check for **contra-indications** or **allergies**.
- Ensure **bare below the elbows**, and **wash hands** (see Chapter 6).
- Collect equipment, including:
  - Non-sterile gloves
  - Water-based lubricant
  - Paper towels.
- Put on **non-sterile gloves**.
- Ask patient to roll onto their **side**, usually the left lateral position (Figure 29.3).
- Part the buttocks, and **inspect** the anus.
- **Lubricate** index finger with water-based lubricant.
- **Warn patient**, and then gently insert the gloved lubricated finger (Figure 29.4).
- Ask the patient to squeeze to **check anal tone**.
- **Rotate** your finger **180° anti-clockwise** to examine the left and anterior side of the pelvis. Assess the prostate gland in men and the pouch of Douglas in females.
- **Rotate** the finger **180°** in the **opposite direction** to examine the right side of the pelvis.
- Perform a bimanual palpation by placing the non-dominant hand on the lower abdomen and palpating for masses between the hands gently.
- Remove finger, and **inspect** any stool or blood on fingertip after removal.
- Provide patient with paper towel to remove any remaining lubricant.
- **Remove gloves**, dispose of waste in clinical waste bins and **wash hands**.
- **Document** in the patient's notes the findings, date, time, signature and designation; any difficulties encountered; the presence of a chaperone; and any additional required information.
- **Thank patient**, and ensure that they are comfortable and have no adverse effects.

Aspects of digital rectal examinations

Inspection of the back passage may reveal pathology such as **anal fissures** (mucosal tears), **anal fistulae** (epithelialised tracks that connect an abscess in the anus or rectum with the skin) and **haemorrhoids** (swellings containing enlarged and swollen blood vessels in or around the rectum and anus).

The **prostate** should be palpable in males – a normal prostate feels flat and smooth, whilst a malignant prostate feels hard and irregular. It may be benignly enlarged in cases of benign prostatic hypertrophy (BPH).

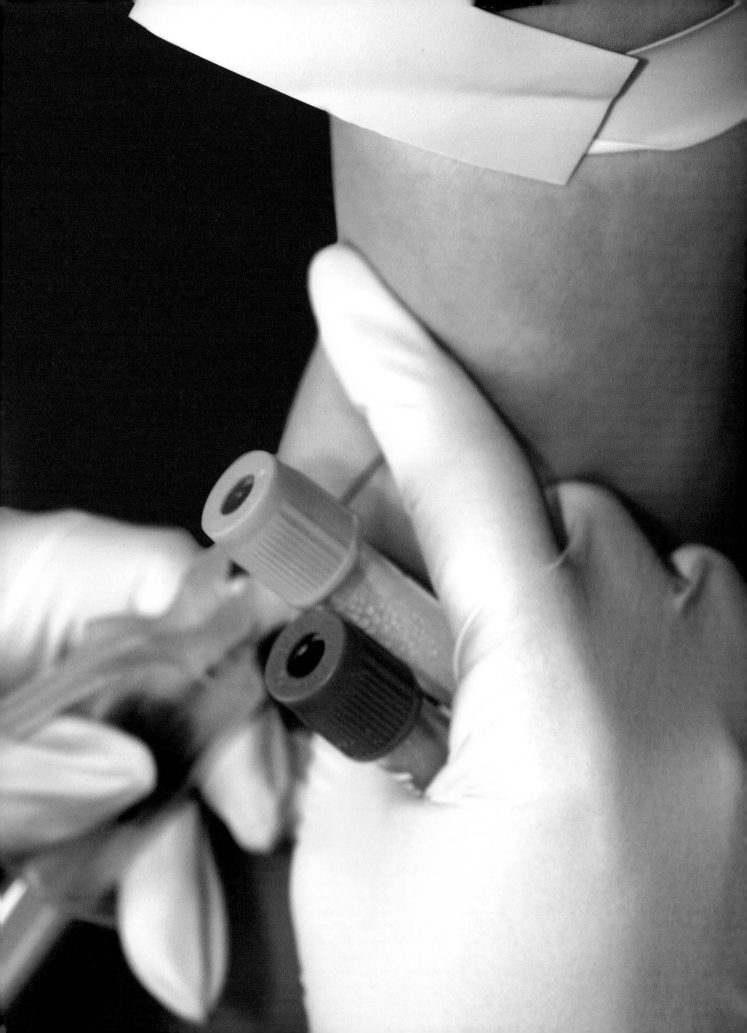

Common procedures – urology

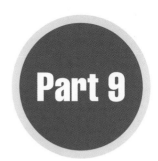

Part 9

Chapters

30   Performing urinalysis   76
31   Inserting a bladder catheter   78

30 Performing urinalysis

Figure 30.1 (a) Collect urine specimen; (b) dip test strip in urine; (c) time according to instructions; (reproduced from iStock © robuart) (d) compare test strip to chart

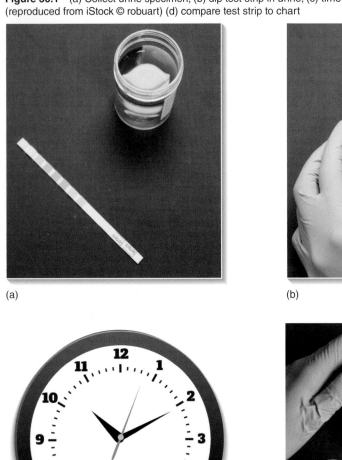

(a)

(b)

(c)

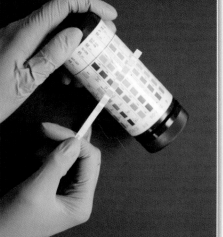

(d)

What is urinalysis?

Urinalysis is a simple test used in clinical practice. It is also referred to as 'urine dip' or 'dipstick' testing. A strip containing a number of **different coloured pads** is dipped in the urine, and then compared to a chart to determine the presence or absence of different substances (Figure 30.1). The pads change colour depending on the urine contents. It is a simple and reliable test.

Urinalysis can be used in many situations, for example to look for **leukocytes** and **nitrites** (evidence of urinary tract infection (UTI)), to look for **blood** (e.g. if there is a suspicion of kidney stones or glomerulonephritis) or to look for **ketones** (e.g. in diabetes). Pregnancy tests are performed on urine but require specialised test strips.

Why is urinalysis important?

Urinalysis gives information on many parameters, including:
- **Leukocyte esterase**: present in white blood cells. If positive, this may indicate a UTI.
- **Nitrites**: produced by bacterial conversion of endogenous nitrates to nitrites. If present, they may indicate a UTI. Note that not all bacteria are able to produce nitrite, therefore, false negatives occur.
- **Urobilinogen**: present in haemolytic anaemia.
- **Protein**: see the 'Aspects of urinalysis' section.
- **pH**: Normal pH is 4.6–8.0. Normally decreased in metabolic acidosis and increased in metabolic alkalosis.
- **Blood**: see the 'Aspects of urinalysis' section.
- **Specific gravity**: an indication of concentration, high in glycosuria, proteinuria and dehydration. Low if excess fluid intake or renal failure is present.
- **Ketones**: present in diabetes and starvation.
- **Bilirubin**: present in obstructive jaundice and liver disease.
- **Glucose**: present in diabetes.
- **βhCG**: elevated in pregnancy.

It is preferable to test a **midstream urine (MSU)** sample as this type of sample **avoids contamination** with bacterial commensals present on the skin and genitals. MSU can be sent for **culture** and **sensitivity** testing in the investigation of a possible UTI.

Indications
- Fever, confusion, late or irregular menstruation
- Urinary frequency, urgency, dysuria

Contra-indications
- Patient refusal
- Unsuitable or aged sample

Complications
- **Local** – nil
- **Systemic** – false readings in incorrectly timed samples

Procedure
- **Introduce** yourself, and **identify** the patient (see Chapter 4).
- Gain **consent** for the procedure (see Chapter 5), explain **indications** and check for **contraindications** or **allergies**.

To obtain an MSU:
- Instruct the patient to:
  - Wash hands and remove cap from sterile container.
  - Begin to pass urine into the toilet with **foreskin retracted** or **labia parted**.
  - Catch the **middle portion** of urine in the container.
  - Fill the container to three-quarters full.
  - Pass the rest of the urine into the toilet.
  - Wash hands and replace the cap.

Alternatively, a sample can be obtained when a patient is **catheterised** (see Chapter 31). After insertion of the catheter, discard the initial portion of urine, and then collect the next portion. Current best practice is to obtain a specimen from the needle-free valve at the catheter–bag junction. (Do not use urine from the catheter bag.) This is a catheter specimen of urine (CSU).

Once you have the sample of urine:
- Ensure **bare below the elbows**, **wash hands** (see Chapter 6) and don **gloves**.
- Find the test strips, and check the **expiry date**.
- **Inspect** the urine for **colour** and **turbidity**; check the **odour** (Figure 30.1a).
- **Dip** test strip in urine (Figure 30.1b).
- Remove test strip, shake off excess urine and hold horizontally.
- **Time accurately** (Figure 30.1c).
- Note **results** as compared to chart (Figure 30.1d).
- Dispose of waste in clinical waste bins.
- **Document** the procedure, **record results** and send for **culture** and **sensitivity** testing if appropriate.
- Thank the patient, and **wash hands**.

Aspects of urinalysis

Normal urine is a **straw yellow** colour. **Dark urine** could be due to dehydration or obstructive jaundice (often alongside pale stools). **Cloudy urine** may be due to a UTI.

Red urine could indicate red blood cells (haematuria), medications such as rifampicin or beetroot ingestion. **Haematuria** may be due to bleeding anywhere in the renal tract – causes can be classified anatomically from the kidney to the genitals, such as renal cell carcinoma, ureteric stones, bladder cancer or UTI. It may be **microscopic** (invisible but detected on a dipstick test) or **macroscopic** (visible).

Frothy urine suggests proteinuria. Healthy adults excrete **<150 mg** protein per day. **Proteinuria** can be transient or persistent. **Transient** causes include exercise, fever, UTI and orthostatic (postural) proteinuria. **Persistent** causes include glomerular and tubular diseases, diabetic nephropathy and pre-eclampsia. A urine dipstick detects **albumin** but not other proteins (hence, it is not a good test for myeloma). Urine that tests positive for protein (proteinuria) on a dipstick should be sent for **albumin–creatinine ratio** testing for quantification.

Did you know?
False positives for **haematuria** may occur from **menstrual blood** or **myoglobin**.

31 Inserting a bladder catheter

Figure 31.1 Urethral catheter (balloon inflated)

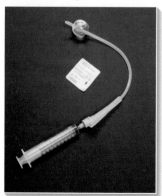

Figure 31.2 Catheter bag

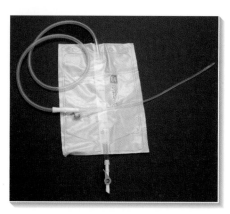

Figure 31.3 Different bladder catheter and local anaesthetic gel sizes

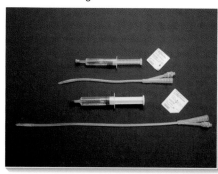

Figure 31.4 Equipment for catheterisation

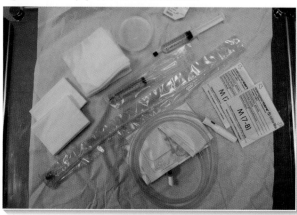

Did you know?

You must always **document** in the notes after catheterising a patient. Things to include are:
- Date, time, designation, bleep number
- Reason for procedure
- Details of catheter used (or place sticker from packet in the notes) (Figures 31.1 and 31.3)
- Aseptic technique used
- Amount of lubricant
- Volume of water used to inflate balloon
- Any problems encountered
- Any complications noted
- Residual volume drained.

Figure 31.5 Catheter insertion into a male

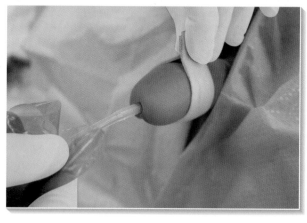

Figure 31.6 Catheter insertion into a female

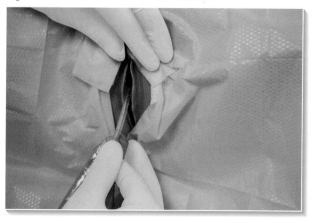

What is bladder catheterisation?

Bladder catheterisation is a procedure during which a plastic catheter (Figure 31.1), attached to a catheter bag (Figure 31.2), is inserted via the urethra into the bladder in order to drain the urine. There are two lengths of catheter: **short (female patients only)** or **standard**, which can be used for **both male and female**

patients (Figure 31.3). The commonest catheter types are **two-way Foley** catheters. **Three-way** catheters can be used for bladder irrigation after surgery to the bladder or prostate.

Catheter size and diameter are measured in **Charrières**, **French gauge** or simply **French** sizes. '1 French' is equivalent to a diameter of one-third of a millimetre, and as the French size increases, so

Practical Medical Procedures at a Glance, First Edition. Rachel K. Thomas © Rachel K. Thomas. Published 2015 by John Wiley & Sons, Ltd.
Companion website: http://www.ataglanceseries.com/practicalmedprocedures

does the diameter (unlike needle gauges!). Usually for a female, you would use a 10–12 French, and for a male you would use 12–14 French. Check the packet carefully for the size and type of catheter you are using, and record this in the notes after the procedure.

Patients with certain chronic conditions requiring catheterisation for spastic bladders can be taught 'in-out' catheterisation, thus avoiding bags and minimising infection risks.

Alternatively, a suprapubic catheter is inserted into the bladder via the abdomen rather than the urethra. This is used in specialised circumstances. Their insertion is beyond the scope of this book.

Why is bladder catheterisation important?

Catheterisation is a common procedure in hospitals. Bladder catheters are also used in conditions where monitoring of fluid balance is needed, such as with the acutely ill in intensive care, in pancreatitis cases, peri-operatively and for retention of urine. Incontinence is **not** an indication for catheterisation except in extreme circumstances to ease nursing. Bladder catheterisation accounts for approximately 30% of healthcare-associated infections; thus, good technique is imperative to minimise this.

Indications
- Surgical procedures, fluid balance monitoring in unwell patients
- Urinary retention (acute and chronic)

Contra-indications
- Traumatic injury to urethra, urethral stricture
- Patient refusal

Complications
- **Local** – urethral trauma strictures, perforation, bleeding, infection
- **Systemic** – infection

Procedure

The procedure can be thought of in two halves: the first half involves preparation of equipment and cleaning of the genital area, and the second half is the insertion of the catheter. Steps specific to males are shown in *italics*.

Part 1
- **Introduce** yourself, and **identify** the patient (see Chapter 4).
- Gain **consent** for the procedure (see Chapter 5), explain **indications** and check for **contra-indications** or **allergies**.
- **Ensure that the patient is socially clean.**
- Ensure **bare below the elbows**, and **wash hands** (see Chapter 6).
- Wipe clean a **trolley** with antibacterial wipes.
- Collect equipment (Figure 31.4), and place it on a trolley using the **aseptic non-touch technique (ANTT)** (see Chapter 8), including:
  - Catheter and catheter bag
  - Antiseptic and anaesthetic lubricating gel
  - Sterile pack containing swabs and drapes
  - Sterile gloves ×2
  - Sterile water
  - Chlorhexidine wipes
  - Water-filled syringe for inflating the balloon.

- Open **sterile pack**, and prepare equipment using **ANTT**. Clean the edge of the package of sterile water with chlorhexidine wipe before opening it, and pour sterile water into dish.
- Position patient supine with external genitalia uncovered. *Males: retract the foreskin; the area must be socially cleaned before the start of the procedure.*
- **Wash hands**, and **put gloves on**.
- Place **sterile drapes** around genitalia, to preserve dignity.
- Perform **aseptic clean**: dip a swab in sterile water. Wipe around urethral meatus (starting from the middle and moving outwards), discarding wipe after each clean. Wash three times.
- Insert **anaesthetic gel (warn patient of stinging sensation)**:
  - *11 ml for males*
  - *6 ml for females*
- **Gel will take 3 to 5 minutes to take effect.**
- Remove gloves, and **wash hands**.
- **Don sterile gloves**.

Part 2
- **Attach** drain to **catheter bag** to ensure a closed system.
- Remove the tip of the catheter from the plastic wrapping, leaving the rest of the catheter in the wrapping (which gives you something to hold without contaminating the catheter itself).
- Place the whole system on the sterile drape between the patient's legs.
- *Hold penis at a 45° angle.* Part the labia with non-dominant hand.
- **Insert** the catheter using the **non-touch technique** (Figures 31.5 and 31.6). As the catheter advances further into the urethra, carefully remove it bit by bit from the plastic wrapping, avoiding touching the catheter itself with your gloved hands.
- When urine begins to drain, continue to insert catheter a further 6 to 10 cm to avoid inflating the balloon in the urethra.
- **Inflate balloon** (usually requires 10–15 ml sterile water).
- **Retract** the catheter gently until you feel a slight resistance, indicating that the balloon is resting against the bladder neck.
- *Replace foreskin.*
- **Check** that urine is draining.
- Tidy up and **secure** the catheter.
- Dispose of waste in clinical waste bins, and clean trolley.
- Remove gloves, and **wash hands**.
- **Attach** the catheter with a **specialised dressing** or **tape** to the **patient's leg**, and **secure drainage bag below the level of the bladder**.
- **Document** in the patient's notes catheter details, date, time, signature, designation, any difficulties encountered and required additional information.
- **Thank patient**, and ensure that they are comfortable and have no adverse effects.

Hints and tips:

In males:
- **Always** replace the foreskin after catheterisation: failure to do this may result in paraphimosis.
- If the catheter fails to pass the prostate, gently apply traction to the penis and change the angle from 45° to zero (0°) whilst at the same time passing the catheter. **Do not force. Do not persist with a bigger size. Ask for senior help before trauma or a false passage is caused.**

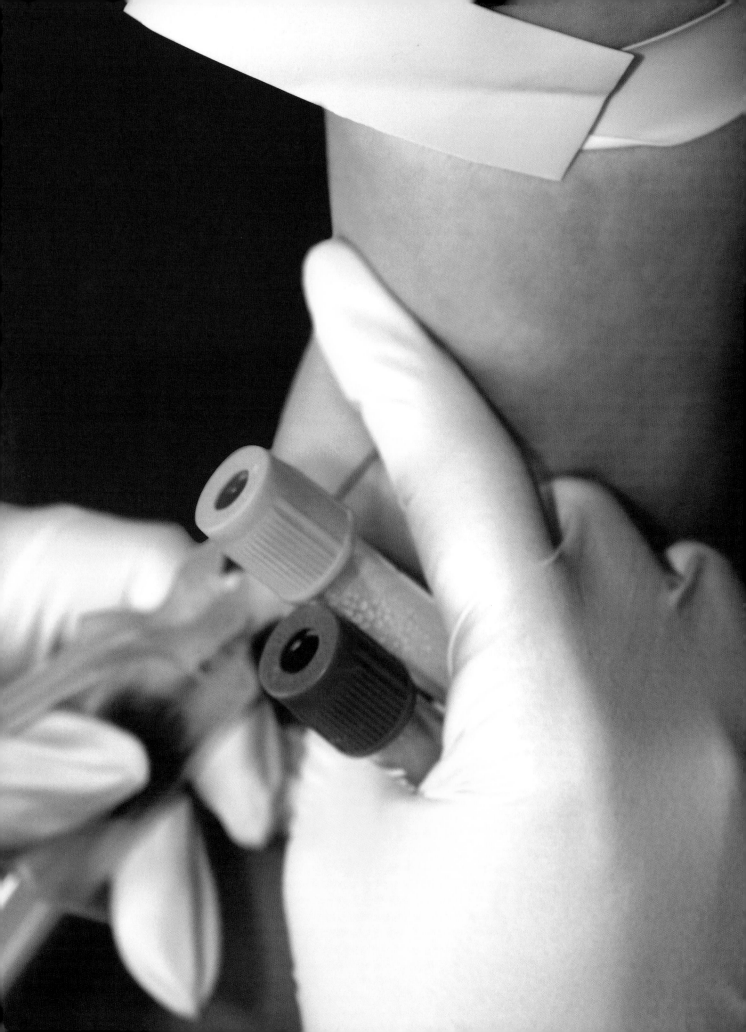

Common procedures – otolaryngology

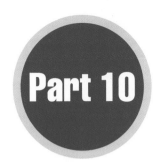

Part 10

Chapter

32 Performing otoscopy 82

32 Performing otoscopy

Figure 32.1 An otoscope

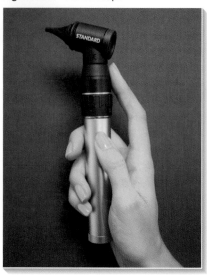

Figure 32.2 Performing otoscopy

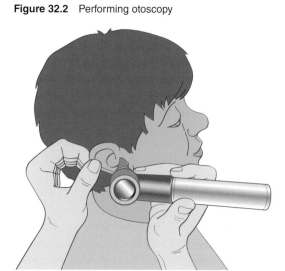

Figure 32.3 Possible findings. Source for (a): Blundell and Harrison (2013), Chapter 112, p. 238. Source for (b), (c) and (d): Blundell and Harrison (2013), Chapter 115, p. 242.

(a) Normal tympanic membrane

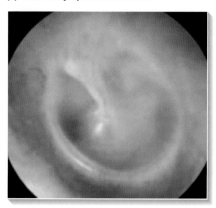

(b) Otisis media

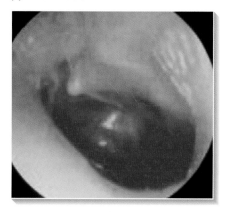

(c) Grommet

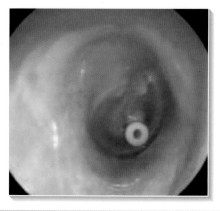

(d) Perforated tympanic membrane

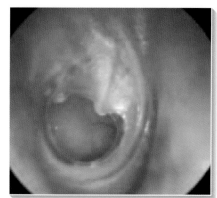

What is otoscopy?

Otoscopy is a technique in which the external ear canal and the tympanic membrane (ear drum) can be **seen**. It is performed using an **otoscope** (Figure 32.1) – a handheld device with a light source, a magnifying lens and a disposable single-use earpiece used to avoid the spread of infection.

Why is otoscopy important?

Otoscopy is performed to investigate **symptoms of ear disease**, such as hearing loss, vertigo (spinning sensation or dizziness), tinnitus (ringing in the ear), otorrhoea (discharge from the ear), otalgia (pain in the ear) and facial weakness.

Indications
- Foreign body
- Investigation of hearing loss or symptoms of ear disease

Contra-indications
- Patient refusal

Complications
- **Local** – local discomfort
- **Systemic** – nil

Procedure

Holding the otoscope:
- Hold the otoscope in your **right hand** to examine the **right ear** and in your **left hand** to examine the **left ear**.
- Hold it like a **pen** (Figure 32.2) with your little finger resting on the patient's cheek and the handle pointing away from the ear.
- Hold the handle near the earpiece.

Performing otoscopy:
- **Introduce** yourself, and **identify** the patient (see Chapter 4).
- Gain **consent** for the procedure (see Chapter 5), explain **indications** and check for **contra-indications**.
- Ensure **bare below the elbows**, and **wash hands** (see Chapter 6).
- Place a new **disposable cap** on the otoscope, using the biggest earpiece that will fit the patient's ear.
- **Sit** the patient comfortably in a chair.
- First, **inspect** around the ear for scars and erythema.
- Next, approach the ear canal with the otoscope, whilst gently pulling the ear **upwards** and **backwards**.

- In children, the ear is pulled **horizontally backwards** (due to the different shape of their ear canal).
- Inspect the external auditory meatus, then gently insert the otoscope until the tympanic membrane is visualised.
- Look for the **light reflex**. Check the **colour** of the membrane. You should be able to see the handle of the malleus. Look for any pathology.
- Check each ear in turn.
- **Thank patient**, and ensure that they are comfortable and have no adverse effects.
- **Dispose** of the disposable cap in the clinical waste bins.
- **Wash hands**.
- **Document** findings in the patient's notes date, time, signature, designation and any difficulties encountered, specifically commenting on the pinna, surrounding structures, canal and drum, and any additional findings.

Aspects of otoscopy

A normal eardrum is almost translucent and appears pink-grey in colour (Figure 32.3a). You should be able to see the **light reflex**, as well as the **handle of the malleus**, and the **umbo** (tip of the handle of the malleus). Look at the shape of the eardrum: normally, it is slightly convex. A very red and/or **bulging** eardrum (suggestive of increased middle ear pressure) may indicate acute otitis media (Figure 32.3b). An eardrum that is **retracted inwards** suggests negative middle ear pressure, and may be found in otitis media with effusion (glue ear). Look for any **grommets**, which are small white plastic ventilation tubes inserted into the tympanic membrane to treat glue ear (Figure 32.3c). Check that they are in the correct position and are patent if present. Look for any **perforations** in the tympanic membrane (Figure 32.3d). An unsafe perforation – such as one in the attic – should be referred to the Ear, Nose and Throat (ENT) team.

Did you know?
Some drugs can cause **hearing loss**, including:
- Loop diuretics (e.g. furosemide)
- Aminoglycoside antibiotics (e.g. vancomycin)
- Salicylates (e.g. aspirin)
- Antimetabolites (e.g. methotrexate).

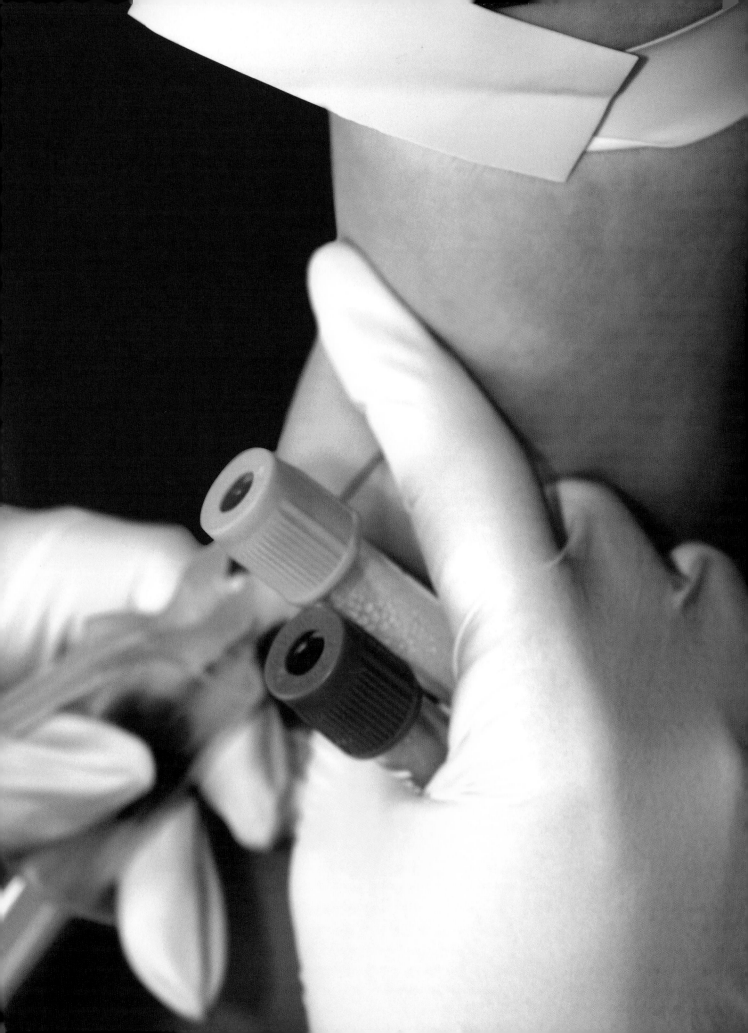

Common procedures – ophthalmology

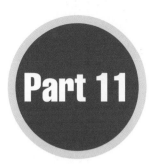

Part 11

Chapter

33   **Performing ophthalmoscopy**   86

33 Performing ophthalmoscopy

Figure 33.1 The ophthalmoscope

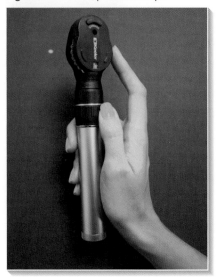

Figure 33.2 Administering dilating eyedrops

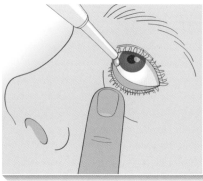

Figure 33.3 Performing ophthalmoscopy

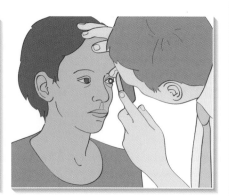

Figure 33.4 Possible findings. Source: Gleadle (2012), Chapter 25, p. 58.

(a) Normal retina

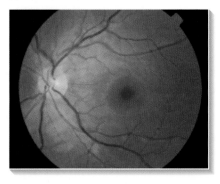

(b) Papilloedema

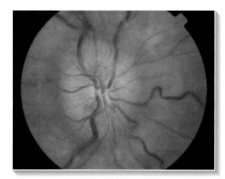

(c) Background diabetic retinopathy

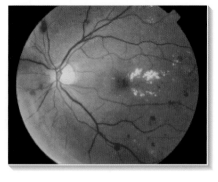

(d) Hypertensive retinopathy

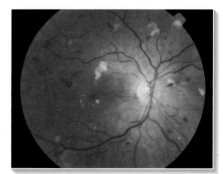

Practical Medical Procedures at a Glance, First Edition. Rachel K. Thomas © Rachel K. Thomas. Published 2015 by John Wiley & Sons, Ltd.
Companion website: http://www.ataglanceseries.com/practicalmedprocedures

What is ophthalmoscopy?

Ophthalmoscopy is a detailed examination of the back of the eye (retina) using a direct **ophthalmoscope** (Figure 33.1), which acts like a magnifying glass to view the anatomy. It is also referred to as **fundoscopy**. It is an important part of any **neurological exam**. It may be necessary to **dilate** the pupil to view the retina. This is often done with **0.5% tropicamide**, an antimuscarinic drug delivered in the form of eye drops (Figure 33.2). This **dilates** the pupil by paralysing the **ciliary muscle**, with a half-life of 4 to 6 hours – thus, patients **should not drive** for several hours while their vision is affected. Rarely, tropicamide can cause acute angle-closure glaucoma, which is an emergency.

Why is ophthalmoscopy important?

Ophthalmoscopy provides information on both **systemic conditions** and **ocular disorders**. For instance, signs of raised intracranial pressure must be excluded in headache presentations; diabetics and hypertensives may have signs of retinopathy. It is also important in the investigation of causes of visual loss, and it can help diagnose conditions such as cataracts, glaucoma, macular degeneration, retinal haemorrhage and retinal detachment.

Indications
- Part of a neurological exam
- Investigation of vision loss, eye pain, headaches

Contra-indications
- Glaucoma – do not use dilating drops
- Patient refusal

Complications
- **Local** – acute angle-closure glaucoma, local discomfort
- **Systemic** – nil

Procedure

Adjusting the ophthalmoscope:
- Patients are best examined in a darkened room.
- Do not remove your own glasses or contact lenses. Set the ophthalmoscope to zero, and adjust it to the patient's prescription. Adjust to their eyesight using the adjustment wheel.
  - – Lenses (usually red numbers) correct for myopia.
  - + Lenses (usually black numbers) correct for hypermetropia.

Performing ophthalmoscopy:
- **Introduce** yourself, and **identify** the patient (see Chapter 4).
- Gain **consent** for the procedure (see Chapter 5), explain **indications** and check for **contra-indications** or **allergies**.
- Ensure **bare below the elbows**, and **wash hands** (see Chapter 6).
- Position patient in a **chair**.
- Administer dilating eye drops, if required, and allow time for these to take effect.

- Ask the patient to fix their **gaze** at a **distant object**, and dim the lights.
- First, check the **red reflex**: shine the ophthalmoscope in each eye in turn from an arm's length away.
- Check and comment on the **anterior structures** of the eye (e.g. the lens).
- Check the **retina**. You should use your right eye to examine the patient's right eye, and your left eye to examine the patient's left. It may help if you place your hand on the patient's forehead (Figure 33.3).
- Try to examine the **optic disc** and the four quadrants of the eye around it (Figure 33.4a).
- Finish by examining the **macula** and **fovea**.
- Check each eye in turn.
- **Thank patient**, and ensure that they are comfortable and have no adverse effects.
- **Wash hands**.
- **Document** findings in the patient's notes, including date, time, signature, designation and any difficulties encountered, specifically commenting on the red reflex, optic disc including colour, cupping and vessels and any additional findings.

Aspects of ophthalmoscopy

Use a structured approach, and develop a routine. Prior to approaching the patient, comment on the **red reflex**. This may be absent due to conditions such as cataracts, the most common cause of vision loss worldwide. Inspect the optic disc – its size, colour, cup–disc ratio and margins – and for new vessels. This may reveal pathology – a pale and clearly demarcated disc may indicate **optic atrophy**, cupping may indicate **glaucoma** and a blurry disc with a yellow colour may be **papilloedema** (Figure 33.4b).

It may help to start at the disc and follow the vessels out, looking for hypertensive and arteriosclerotic changes. Look as far as the mid-periphery for scars (e.g. inflammatory, laser), haemorrhages, exudates and pigment. Look for signs of **diabetic retinopathy** (Figure 33.4c). Flame haemorrhages are a sign of hypertensive retinopathy (Figure 33.4d).

The **macula** is temporal to the disc, and it can be seen best with the patient looking **directly** into the light of the ophthalmoscope. A normal macula is a darker area approximately 2.5 mm in diameter. A cherry-red macula is a sign of arterial obstruction.

Hints and tips:
Don't be afraid to get really **close** to the patient! A common reason for failing to see the optic disc is being too far away.
- When you identify a blood vessel, use it to guide you towards the optic disc.
- Don't use **dilating eye drops** for patients with **glaucoma**.
- If drops are used, advise patients that their vision will **blur** for several hours after administration.

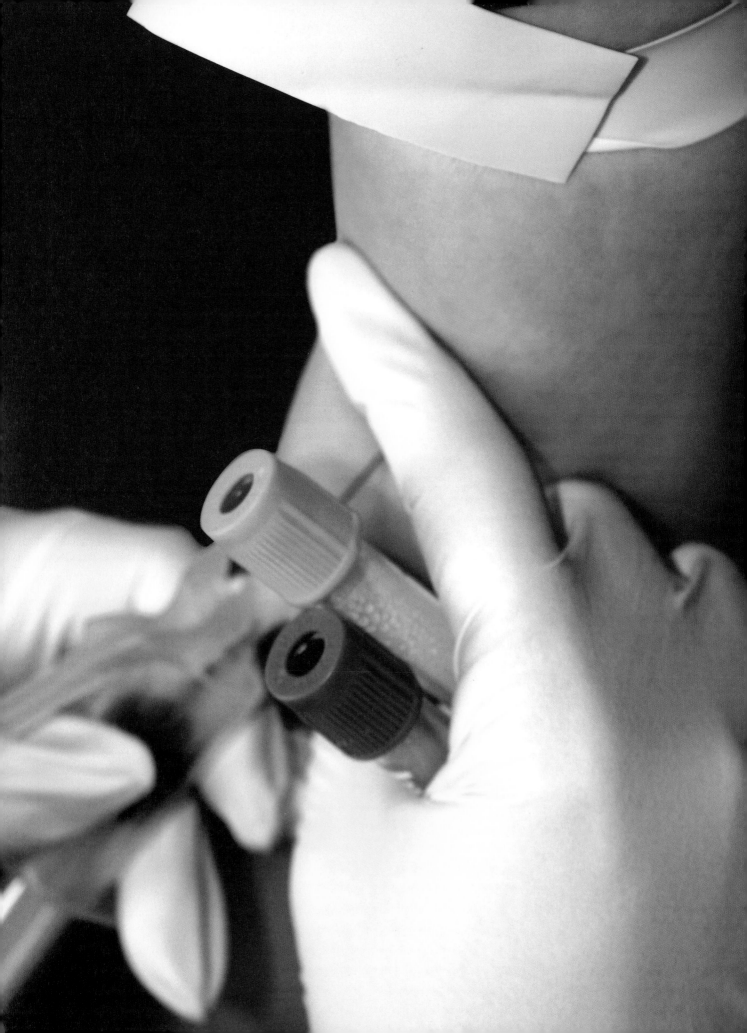

Common procedures – end-of-life care

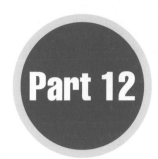

Part 12

Chapter

34 **Confirming and certifying death** 90

34 Confirming and certifying death

Figure 34.1 Confirming death

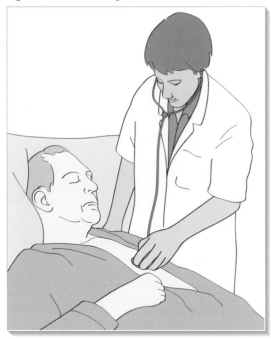

Figure 34.2 Documentation in notes

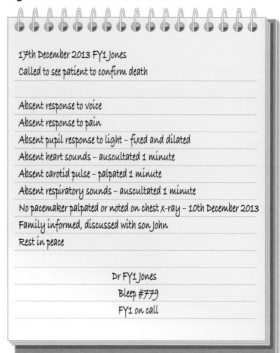

17th December 2013 FY1 Jones
Called to see patient to confirm death

Absent response to voice
Absent response to pain
Absent pupil response to light – fixed and dilated
Absent heart sounds – auscultated 1 minute
Absent carotid pulse – palpated 1 minute
Absent respiratory sounds – auscultated 1 minute
No pacemaker palpated or noted on chest x-ray – 10th December 2013
Family informed, discussed with son John
Rest in peace

Dr FY1 Jones
Bleep #779
FY1 on call

Hints and tips:
- Ask family members to leave the room whilst diagnosing death.
- Ask for **senior help** if you are unclear of the cause of death.
- Ensure you record the **cause** of death, not the mode.
- While it is preferable to attend to the patient promptly, this diagnosis is generally **not urgent**.
- Some sounds may still be heard on auscultation – **fluid** settling in the lungs, some **gastric noises** – if you are unsure, request an **ECG**.
- Chest X-rays and previous ECGs can be used for detecting **pacemakers**.

Figure 34.3 Example of a death certificate

25. PART 1. Enter the diseases, injuries, or complications that caused the death. Do not enter the mode of dying, such as cardiac or respiratory arrest, shock, or heart failure. List only one cause on each line.	Approximate interval Between Onset and Death
IMMEDIATE CAUSE (Final disease or condition resulting in death) — a. CARDIOPULMONARY ARREST	MINUTES
DUE TO (OR AS A CONSEQUENCE OF): b. ASPIRATION EVENT	18 HOURS
DUE TO (OR AS A CONSEQUENCE OF): c. VOMITTING	18 HOURS
DUE TO (OR AS A CONSEQUENCE OF): d. PNEUMONIA	2 DAYS

PART 2. Other significant conditions contributing to death but not resulting in the underlying cause given in Part 1. DIABETES MELLITUS

25a. DID TOBACCO USE CONTRIBUTE TO DEATH? ☐Yes ☐Probably ☑No ☐Unknown | 25b. WAS AN AUTOPSY PERFORMED ☐Yes ☑No | 26c. WERE AUTOPSY FINDINGS AVAILABLE PRIOR TO COMPLETION OF CAUSE OF DEATH ☐Yes ☐No

27a. MANNER OF DEATH ☑Natural ☐Accident ☐Suicide ☐Homicide ☐Undet. ☐Pending | 27b. DATE OF INJURY | 27c. HOUR | 27d. HOW DID THE INJURY OCCUR

27e. INJURY AT WORK | 27f. PLACE OF INJURY | 27g. LOCATION

Practical Medical Procedures at a Glance, First Edition. Rachel K. Thomas © Rachel K. Thomas. Published 2015 by John Wiley & Sons, Ltd.
Companion website: http://www.ataglanceseries.com/practicalmedprocedures

What is confirming and certifying death?

Death is confirmed when an **absence of vital signs** is formally observed and recorded (Figure 34.1). This needs to be **documented** in the patient's notes (Figure 34.2). In more complex cases, such as those involving brain death and organ transplantation, senior physicians will be responsible for using other criteria and tests in order to diagnose death.

Deaths need to be **certified** and then **registered** with the **Registrar of Births and Deaths**. Before a death can be **registered** with the Registrar of Births and Deaths, a **medical practitioner** must issue a **Medical Certificate of the Cause of Death (MCCD)** (Figure 34.3). This can be done only if they have seen the patient in the last **14 days** and there were no **unnatural**, **suspicious** or **unknown causes** involved in the death. In cases where these or other factors are suspected, the death must be referred to **Her Majesty's (HM) Coroner**, who may investigate further to determine the **cause** of death. (Note that in England, Northern Ireland and Wales, the referrals are made to HM Coroner, while in Scotland they are made to the Procurator Fiscal.)

Why is confirming and certifying death important?

Death needs to be confirmed to enable the **bereavement process** for the patient's next of kin and family to begin. If family members are present when you see the patient, they may have questions on aspects of the death, and what will happen next. It is advisable to familiarise yourself with the **patient's history** prior to meeting them, if you have not been previously involved with the patient. After death, the patient is transferred to the **mortuary** until collection for the funeral.

The MCCD has different **sections** which need to be completed **accurately**, **legibly** and **without abbreviations** (Figure 34.3). Always **confirm** the information with a senior prior to beginning the MCCD, as what is recorded can influence aspects such as **compensation**.

Section 1a) refers to the **specific condition** that **caused** the death of the patient. It must be a **cause** of death, such as myocardial infarction, **not a mode**, such as collapse. **Section 1b)**, **Section 1c)** and **Section 1d)** refer to other diseases present which may have **caused** or **significantly contributed** to Section 1a). It may be acceptable on occasions to leave Section 1b) to 1d) **blank**, but not Section 1a).

Section 2) refers to **other disease processes** that may have contributed to the death, but did not directly cause it.

Other sections such as the **patient's name**, **date of birth** and **address**, and the **doctor's name**, **signature**, **designation** and **qualifications**, also need to be completed. Part of this information needs to be **rewritten** on another small section of the certificate, which remains in the hospital records, while the main certificate is given to the patient's next of kin, who lodge it with the Registrar of Births and Deaths. In the absence of next of kin, the signing doctor must ensure that the certificate reaches the Registrar. The Registrar then issues another certificate once the death has been **formally registered**.

In some cases, the MCCD cannot be completed. These include cases where the cause of death is **unknown**, **unnatural** or **suspicious**, and these should be referred **as soon as possible** to HM **Coroner**. Deaths **caused by medical intervention**, **violence** or **neglect**, or **within 24 hours** of having been admitted to hospital prior to a diagnosis being made, should be referred. If unsure, seek senior advice or contact the HM Coroner's office directly for assistance. General Medical Council and National Health Service guidance is also readily available. HM Coroner may hold **further** investigations such as an **autopsy** (post-mortem examination) before then issuing a **certificate** if appropriate.

Procedure

- **Identify** the patient (see Chapter 4).
- Ensure **bare below the elbows**, and **wash hands** (see Chapter 6).
- **Don gloves**.
- Check for an **absence of response to voice** by speaking the patient's name clearly into each ear, and ask them to respond to you.
- Check for an **absence of response to pain** by rubbing the patient's sternum with a moderate pressure.
- Check for **absence of pupil response** by shining light in each eye from a pen torch.
- Check for **absence of heart sounds** by auscultating the praecordium for at least 1 minute.
- Check for **absence of circulation** by palpating the carotid pulse for at least 1 minute.
- Check the left sub-clavicular region for the presence of a **pacemaker**.
- Check for **absence of breath sounds** by auscultating the chest for at least 1 minute.
- Remove gloves, and **wash hands**.
- **Record** in the patient's notes the **time** and **date** of **confirmation** of death.
- **Record signature**, **name** and **designation**.
- **Record** if family members were present and what they were told.

Aspects of confirming and certifying death

Most Healthcare Trusts have **support services** to facilitate both patients and doctors during difficult circumstances such as death. **Bereavement officers** are able to help **co-ordinate** paperwork, acting as a single point where relatives can collect **information**, **documents** and **belongings**. They can often provide **counselling**, and assist in finding other services to help with funeral arrangements. They are **experts** at this sensitive time, and thus requesting their help is advisable as this can be a difficult time for families and next of kin. The Bereavement Office also liaises with different departments within the hospital, including the mortuary and pathology.

It is advisable to contact the patient's **General Practitioner (GP)** to inform them of the death and its causes.

A **Cremation Form** must be completed prior to a patient's release for cremation. These forms are a **legal document**, verifying the patient's **identity** and an **absence** of a **pacemaker** or other specific implants. Pacemakers can be detected by checking the patient's notes, and by palpation and chest X-rays, or by looking for pacing spikes on old electrocardiograms. You receive a **sum** for completing the form, as it is beyond the 'regular requirements' of most jobs – if accepted, this sum needs to be included in your **income** for tax purposes.

Did you know?

Some causes of death must be referred to **HM Coroner**, such as:
- Suspicious or violent circumstances
- Suicides or neglect
- Unknown or unnatural causes
- Drug related
- Industry related
- Due to medical procedures or interventions
- Less than 24 hours after admission to hospital
- Not seen by a doctor in the 14 days prior to death.

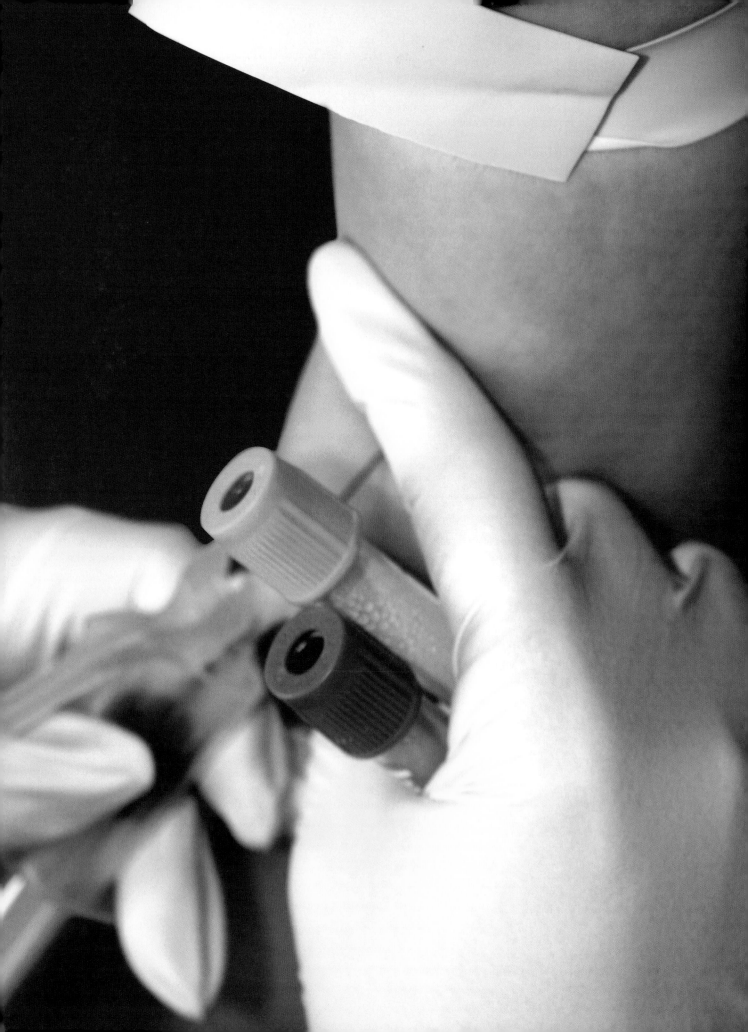

Supplementary resources

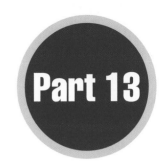

Part 13

Resources

Multiple choice questions 94
Answers to multiple choice questions 104
Further reading and references 114

Multiple choice questions

1 Overview of practical procedures

1 Proficiency in practical procedures is:
   A required for quality patient care
   B sometimes useful
   C rarely useful
   D encouraged but not a recommendation

2 Practical procedures are used:
   A daily in most hospitals
   B to aid in the diagnosis of conditions
   C to monitor the treatment of conditions
   D all of the above

3 If you are unsure of how to perform a procedure:
   A guess
   B attempt it
   C seek senior help
   D request a different procedure and pretend you didn't want the original one

4 In some situations, some practical procedures may be performed by:
   A porters
   B nursing staff
   C relatives
   D patients

5 As a medical professional, it is your responsibility to:
   A ensure that you keep up with 'best current practice'
   B adhere to local policies and procedures
   C ensure you do no harm to the patient
   D all of the above

2 Non-technical skills

1 Communication includes:
   A spoken words
   B actions
   C written words and diagrams
   D all of the above

2 When communicating, it is good practice to:
   A minimise eye contact
   B use family members as translators
   C have a relaxed yet attentive posture
   D discuss patients whenever and wherever it suits you

3 Task management involves prioritising activities:
   A in order of ease
   B in order of importance
   C in order of difficulty
   D in order of duration

4 Situation awareness involves:
   A asking questions to maximise understanding
   B anticipating what may occur
   C interpreting information
   D all of the above

5 Teamwork involves:
   A telling people what to do
   B an awareness of both your and your teammates' capabilities and limitations
   C minimal communication
   D ignoring allocated roles

3 Waste, sharps disposal and injuries

1 Clinical waste bins are commonly:
   A green
   B black
   C blue
   D yellow

2 Confidential waste should be disposed of in:
   A recycling bins
   B confidential waste bins
   C clinical waste bins
   D clinical sharps bins

3 With regards to sharps, you should:
   A never re-sheathe one
   B use a needle-safe unit after use if one is present
   C dispose of them as soon as possible in a dedicated clinical sharps bin
   D all of the above

4 If a sharps injury occurs:
   A ignore it
   B simply cover it with a sterile dressing
   C encourage bleeding and contact occupational health
   D confront the patient regarding any illnesses they may have

5 Clinical waste to be disposed of in a yellow clinical waste bin includes:
   A food wrappers
   B soiled incontinence products
   C patient wristbands
   D drafts of patient referrals

4 Identifying a patient

1 Patients must be:
   A identified at the start of each clinical encounter
   B identified using multiple data points
   C wearing a wristband if they are an inpatient
   D all of the above

2 Incorrect identification of a patient is:
   A advisable
   B a 'never event'
   C permitted on occasion
   D easily forgiven

3 In order to ascertain a patient's identity, they should be asked:
   A 'Are you Mrs Jones?'
   B 'Can you please tell me your full name?'

C nothing, if you have already been told their name

D nothing, if it is written above or near their hospital bed

4 Studies of hospital errors have shown that:

A half were preventable

B a quarter were preventable

C none were preventable

D all were preventable

5 Patient safety rights include ensuring that the right patient:

A is given the right treatment

B is given the right dose, through the right route

C has treatment administered at the right time

D all of the above

5 Consent, capacity and documentation

1 Consent should be:

A forced

B pre-arranged

C voluntary

D ignored

2 As part of the *assessment* of capacity, a patient must be able to:

A talk in a socially appropriate manner

B understand the information which is conveyed to them

C consent to a procedure

D refuse a treatment

3 In the assessment of capacity:

A all cases are clear and easily defined

B some cases may be difficult to determine

C you, as the treating clinician, must decide it

D it is regarded as a fixed entity – it is present or not present, and does not change

4 Regarding consent:

A it can later be withdrawn, if a patient has capacity

B it cannot ever be withdrawn, once given

C it is not an important aspect of interventions

D it is only required for a few interventions, such as surgical procedures

5 Regarding consent:

A it can and must be spoken

B it can only be spoken

C it may be implied in some instances

D it must always be written

6 Hand hygiene and personal protective equipment

1 There are how many basic steps in handwashing, and how many moments for hand hygiene?

A 4, 5

B 5, 5

C 5, 6

D 6, 5

2 PPE is short for:

A public protection equipment

B personal protective equipment

C personal production equipment

D public persona equipment

3 Hand hygiene is required:

A only if gloves are not worn

B before putting on gloves only

C after removing gloves only

D before gloves are put on, and after they are removed

4 Alcoholic rubs are:

A the only type of hand hygiene required

B not effective against some bacteria, such as *Clostridium difficile*

C rarely used in hospitals

D used to replace the need for washing with water and an antibacterial agent in all instances

5 Hand hygiene is:

A of little use

B barely noticed

C very important in reducing disease transmission

D good to do on occasion

7 Scrubbing in

1 Scrubbing in is also commonly known as:

A cleaning up

B washing in

C surgical scrubbing

D surgical bathing

2 There are two main types of solution commonly used to scrub in. These are usually:

A pink and brown

B white and clear

C green and blue

D colourless

3 If you touch a non-sterile surface after you have scrubbed in, prior to the procedure starting:

A pretend you did not touch it

B do not worry if it was only a quick touch

C tell someone, and start the scrubbing-in process again as you are no longer sterile

D deny having touched anything

4 Once you have scrubbed in for theatre, and you are moving around the theatre, but the procedure has not yet commenced:

A move normally around the theatre

B it is acceptable to readjust your cap, shoes and mask

C it is acceptable to touch any items

D move carefully around the theatre, with your hands carefully in front of you, touching nothing that is not also sterile

5 During the first few sessions when you scrub in:

A prepare well, collect your equipment in advance and take your time

B be quick so that you do not delay the theatre list

C collect equipment as you need it, not before, so as not to waste it

D don't worry if you contaminate yourself, as there is no need to start again

8 Asepsis

1 The aseptic technique, also referred to as the aseptic non-touch technique (ANTT), aims to:

A minimise the possibility of infectious contamination

B complicate procedures

C replace handwashing

D prolong procedures

2 ANTT should be used for:

A chest drain insertion

B wound care

C bladder catheterisation

D all of the above

3 Key sites are:

A areas of pain in the body

B sites in the body through which infection may be introduced during a procedure

C areas requiring locking in the patient

D not important to identify

4 A key part is:

A a part of a piece of equipment which, if contaminated, may introduce infection into a key site

B a part of a piece of equipment which is easily broken and is thus important

C a piece of equipment which is not important to recognise

D not important

5 Key parts include:

A the catheter tip

B the saline flush syringe top

C the cannula tip

D all of the above

9 Measuring vital signs

1 Commonly measured vital signs include:

A respiratory rate

B appetite

C mood

D weight

2 Vital signs are useful:

A as an absolute value

B as part of a clinical trend

C as indicators of a patient's state

D all of the above

3 Oxygen saturation can be measured:

A with an inflatable cuff

B in the inner ear

C on the ear lobe

D by auscultation

4 Temperature may be measured:

A in the rectum

B in the ear

C under the tongue

D all of the above

5 When measuring routine vital signs, the pulse is most commonly determined by palpating the:

A radial artery

B femoral artery

C popliteal artery

D abdominal artery

10 Writing a safe prescription

1 When writing a prescription:

A OD, PRN and TDS represent once, twice and three times a day, respectively

B OD, BD and TDS represent once, twice and three times a day, respectively

C OM, TDS and QDS represent once, twice and three times a day, respectively

D ON, PR and PRN represent once, twice and three times a day, respectively

2 Prescriptions should:

A be written in pen

B be legible

C use generic names for medications (unless hospital protocols dictate otherwise for common medications)

D all of the above

3 The fluid status and cardiovascular status should be assessed prior to administration of fluids. Whilst varying significantly with each clinical picture, an elderly, fluid-overloaded patient with cardiovascular disease may require:

A fluids given more slowly than to a healthy, young, elective pre-operative patient

B fluids given at the same speed as to a healthy, young, elective pre-operative patient

C fluids given more quickly than to a healthy, young, elective pre-operative patient

D it doesn't matter

4 Oxygen:

A does not need to be prescribed as it is so commonly administered

B can be prescribed by nursing staff

C should be prescribed as it is a medication, including if it is to be given intermittently or continuously

D saturations always need to be at the same levels, greater than 98%

5 In writing prescriptions, it is generally acceptable to use:

A u for 'units'

B μ for 'micro'

C PRN for 'as required;

D pencil, if a pen is not available

11 Performing venepuncture

1 Veins suitable for venepuncture should be selected by:

A sight

B previous usage

C gentle palpation

D close proximity to an arteriovenous (A-V) fistula

2 A suitable vein may be in:

A an A-V fistula

B a region of cellulitis

C a region of phlebitis

D the ante-cubital fossa

3 A suitable angle and orientation of insertion for the needle are:

A 90°, bevel up

B 60°, bevel down

C less than 45°, bevel up

D less than 45°, bevel down

4 Venepuncture is not useful for helping in:

A monitoring levels of medications

B diagnosis of conditions

C indicating the effects of antibiotics

D any of the above

5 When taking blood, you do not:

A gain consent

B label specimens

C maximise patient comfort

D fill vials in any random order

12   Taking blood cultures

1 In order to take blood cultures, you do not need:

A patient consent

B chlorhexidine wipes

C an electrocardiogram (ECG) tracing

D a clinical indication

2 The main reason to taken an anaerobic sample is:

A to indicate the presence of organisms that require oxygen

B to indicate medication levels

C to indicate the presence of organisms that do not require oxygen

D to indicate patient compliance

3 Anaerobic samples should be taken:

A first

B second

C after other blood samples have been collected

D it doesn't matter

4 Blood culture samples should be sent to:

A Microbiology

B Haematology

C Chemistry

D Biochemistry

5 Blood cultures may be required if:

A there are signs of sepsis

B a patient has a persistently high temperature

C a patient has a spike in temperature

D all of the above

13   Inserting a cannula in a peripheral vein

1 Cannulae may be required for administering:

A blood

B IV fluids

C medications

D all of the above

2 Prior to inserting a cannula, the area should be cleaned with:

A nothing

B chlorhexidine

C socially clean

D soap and water

3 'Primary flashback' is seen:

A in the shaft of the tube as it is advanced

B in the window at the back of the cannula when it is first inserted into the vein

C on the gauze as the cannula is placed

D rarely, and it can be noted in different areas

4 Blood samples can be taken:

A when the cannula is first inserted, and only then

B when the cannula is first inserted, and one other time if the bung is carefully cleaned

C never; the patient needs to be bled elsewhere

D anytime, as long as a Vacutainer® connector collection system is used

5 A preferable vein for cannulation is:

A seen but not felt

B palpable and bendy

C any vein

D palpable and straight

14   Measuring blood glucose

1 Blood glucose measurements:

A are always accurate

B should be checked in the laboratory by a plasma glucose sample

C are slow to obtain and therefore should not be used in emergencies

D are rarely used

2 The lancet used to prick the patient's finger should be disposed of in:

A the clinical waste bin

B the recycling bin

C the clinical sharps bin

D the domestic waste bin

3 When pricking a patient with the lancet to obtain a sample:

A use their thumb

B use the fat on their abdomen, rotating the sites of puncture

C use their antecubital fossa

D use the pulp on the side of a finger

4 A blood glucose measurement may be helpful in the investigation of a patient presenting with:

A confusion

B tremor

C palpitations

D all of the above

5 Prior to using the handheld glucose monitor:

A check the expiry date on the reagent strips

B check the patient's identity

C ensure you have access to a clinical sharps bin

D all of the above

15   Suturing

1 An example of a non-absorbable suture is:

A Monocryl

B Vicryl

C Prolene

D steri-strips

2 Common wound closure methods include:

A sutures and steri-strips

B glue

C staples

D all of the above

3 Prior to suturing, it is advisable to check:

A tetanus status

B name of patient

C neurovascular status of distal region

D all of the above

4 Non-absorbable sutures in the face could be removed (approximately, as this varied with clinical picture) in:

A 1–2 days

B 5–7 days

C 10–12 days

D 15–17 days

5 When suturing, the edges of the skin generally need to be slightly:

A inverted

B everted

C level

D overlapping

16 Administering intravenous infusions

1 Prior to administering the fluids, the cannula always must be:

A reinserted

B flushed

C moved

D replaced

2 For administering:

A Gelofusine®, use a crystalloid giving set

B blood, use a crystalloid giving set

C saline, use a crystalloid giving set

D none of the above

3 'Priming' the line of the giving set means:

A checking the expiration date, strength and name of the medication

B running sterile saline through the entire length of the tube

C giving the medication first

D flicking the edge of the syringe to ensure that no air bubbles are present prior to administration

4 In order to *ensure* a steady delivery rate of the infusion:

A watch the infusion administration in its entirety

B request nursing staff to monitor the patient frequently

C administer it with a pump

D prescribe a fast administration timeframe

5 Prior to attaching the giving set to the cannula:

A touch the key parts

B touch the key sites

C open the roller so that the fluid flows freely

D wipe the end of the cannula or bung with a chlorhexidine wipe

17 Administrating intravenous infusions of blood and blood products

1 A patient's blood group can be determined by:

A a questionnaire asking the group

B asking the patient's relatives for the group

C a blood sample testing for the group

D a blood cultures testing for the group

2 'Universal donor' blood type is:

A A

B B

C AB

D O

3 Patients may:

A refuse blood transfusions if they have capacity

B request blood transfusions if they have capacity but no clinical indication

C demand blood transfusions if they have capacity but no clinical indication

D refuse blood if they do not have capacity

4 Prior to giving the blood transfusion:

A check patient's details and the blood details both with a colleague and at the patient's bedside

B do not worry about checking the patient's details

C do not worry about checking the blood details

D check the details of the patient and blood by yourself only

5 During a transfusion, ensure:

A the patient has plenty to drink

B the patient has their vital signs monitored frequently

C the patient remains completely still

D the patient does not eat

18 Administering parenteral medications

1 When drawing up IV medications:

A a large-gauge needle should be used, to draw it up quickly

B any gauge needle can be used

C a fine-gauge needle should be used, to prevent the uptake of shards of glass

D only medications in pre-packaged administration kits should be used

2 When preparing IV medications:

A ensure thorough mixing prior to administration

B medications mix and distribute themselves adequately and do not need additional mixing

C medications do not require mixing

D a quick shake is adequate

3 Medication doses:

A never vary according to the route of administration

B may vary according to the route of administration

C never vary renal impairment

D never require double-checking with a colleague

4 An IV medication should not be given if:

A the patient has had a previous anaphylactic reaction to it

B the patient is refusing it, and the patient has capacity

C the medication is past its expiry date

D all of the above

5 After administration:

A some medications may require additional monitoring of the patient to be instigated

B of some medications, patients do not need to ever be observed for any adverse signs

C do not worry about any additional monitoring for some medications

D additional 'left over' medication can be replaced into the container it was originally in for later use, as long as the container is still sterile

19 Administering injections

1 After inserting the needle for an injection, and prior to administering the medication:

A aspirate, to ensure you are not in a blood vessel

B inject as quickly as possible

C move the tip of the needle around

D move the site of the injection

2 It is appropriate to inject into:
A a patient who has an allergy to the medication about to be administered
B a region of cellulitis
C a patient who has capacity and is refusing the medication
D a patient who has a clinical indication for the medication and who has agreed to have it

3 Generally speaking, use:
A a large-gauge needle for intradermal (ID) injections, and a fine-gauge needle for intramuscular (IM) ones
B a large-gauge needle for ID, and a large-gauge needle for IM
C a fine-gauge needle for ID, and a large-gauge needle for IM
D a fine-gauge needle for ID, and a fine-gauge needle for IM

4 Intradermal injections are used for:
A systemic delivery of medications
B local delivery of medications
C large, quick-action doses
D slow-delivery doses

5 Generally, the most painful type of injection is:
A intradermal
B subcutaneous
C intramuscular
D intravenous

20 Measuring arterial blood gas

1 To obtain an arterial blood gas, it is preferable to sample in the patient:
A any artery in the ante-cubital fossa
B any vein in the ante-cubital fossa
C the radial artery, non-dominant arm
D the ulnar artery, non-dominant arm

2 When positioning the patient:
A they should be standing
B dorsiflex the wrist
C keep the wrist straight
D elevate the arm

3 Prior to taking an ABG from the radial artery, you should perform:
A a modified Allen test
B a Gillick test
C a Fraser test
D a blood test

4 Prior to analysing a sample:
A expel air bubbles
B agitate the sample
C note patient details, including oxygen therapy concentrations
D all of the above

5 ABG analysis may also indicate:
A Temperature
B Haemoglobin
C Bilirubin
D Respiratory rate

21 Administering oxygen therapy

1 Oxygen therapy is generally always used for patients who are:
A without capacity
B hypoxaemic

C demanding
D sleepy

2 Target oxygen saturations:
A should be not prescribed, and are 94–98% for a healthy adult
B should be prescribed, and are 94–98% for a healthy adult
C should be not prescribed, and are 88–92% for a healthy adult
D should be prescribed, and are 88–92% for a healthy adult

3 The highest percentage of inspired oxygen is delivered by:
A nasal cannulae
B a simple oxygen face mask
C a Venturi mask
D a non-rebreathe mask

4 A high oxygen requirement is a sign of:
A health
B vitality
C illness severity
D prescribing error

5 Oxygen must be:
A prescribed on the medication card
B regarded as a medication
C generally gradually reduced as tolerated and clinically indicated
D all of the above

22 Using inhalers and nebulisers

1 Inhalers and nebulisers:
A are used to deliver medications to the airways
B must be prescribed
C require different amounts of co-ordination
D all of the above

2 If a patient is having difficulty using an inhaler, first you should:
A prescribe a different medication
B consider attaching it to a spacer
C ignore their issue as it is not relevant if they have capacity
D refer them to another doctor

3 If a patient requires a nebuliser but is not comfortable using the mask:
A prescribe them inhalers instead
B check their inhaler technique
C consider using the handheld mouthpiece device
D intubate them

4 Inhalers may:
A contain more than one medication
B be difficult to co-ordinate for some patients
C be used as part of a stepwise treatment program for conditions such as asthma
D all of the above

5 The quantity of medication required for a nebuliser medication chamber is approximately:
A 1–2 ml
B 4–10 ml
C 10–15 ml
D 16–20 ml

23 Assessing respiratory function

1 Peak flow meters measure:
A a person's maximum rate of airflow during a sudden forced expiration starting from full inspiration
B tidal volume
C the differences between restrictive and obstructive diseases
D forced expiratory volume

2 Total lung capacity is measured by:
A spirometry
B a peak flow meter
C plethysmography
D a nebuliser

3 Prior to using a peak flow meter:
A zero the meter by sliding back the indicator to the zero position
B fully identify the patient
C apply a single-use disposable mouthpiece
D all of the above

4 Peak flow readings are particularly helpful in the longer term monitoring of conditions such as:
A lung cancer
B asthma
C flu
D gastritis

5 Peak flow readings vary with:
A age
B gender
C height
D all of the above

24 Using airway manoeuvres and simple adjuncts

1 Airway manoeuvres include:
A jaw thrust, chin tilt and head lift
B head tilt, chin thrust and jaw lift
C head tilt, chin lift and jaw thrust
D head thrust, chin lift and jaw tilt

2 Airway adjuncts include:
A nasopharyngeal airway
B laryngeal mask airway (LMA)
C oropharyngeal airway
D all of the above

3 Unless the benefits outweigh the risks associated with use, nasopharyngeal airways should generally not be used in:
A children
B the elderly
C patients with broken teeth
D patients with a suspected skull base fracture

4 To size an oropharyngeal airway, measure:
A the width of the patient's smallest finger
B from the incisor to the angle of the jaw
C from the lips to the angle of the jaw
D nothing, and always use the same size adjunct for adults

5 Suction should only be used:
A on elderly patients
B under direct vision
C on children
D if instructed by a senior

25 Ventilating with a bag valve mask device

1 A bag valve mask device is most frequently used with:
A only the elderly
B an airway adjunct *in situ*
C hyperventilating patients
D only one hand

2 Bag valve mask devices are generally found:
A in the wet sluice room
B in the medication room
C in the doctors' office
D on the resuscitation trolley

3 When applying the mask to the patient's face:
A hold your thumb only on each side of the mask, and push down firmly
B hold your thumb and index finger in the shape of a 'C' on each side of the mask
C hold your thumb and index finger on one side of the mask, preferably at the top of it
D hold it in a position that the patient finds comfortable

4 Squeezing the bag of the bag valve mask device delivers to the patient:
A nitrous oxide or air
B oxygen or air
C helium or oxygen
D general anaesthetic or air

5 The best way to assess ventilation is with:
A spirometry
B capnography
C X-ray
D a stethoscope

26 Recording a 12-lead electrocardiogram

1 To obtain a 12-lead electrocardiogram, you require:
A six chest leads and six limb leads
B six chest leads and four limb leads
C four chest leads and eight limb leads
D eight chest leads and four limb leads

2 In an ECG, a positive deflection in the ECG waveform reflects:
A depolarisation of the muscle flowing away from the electrode
B repolarisation of the muscle flowing towards the electrode
C depolarisation of the muscle flowing towards the electrode
D repolarisation of the muscle flowing perpendicular to the electrode

3 The paper in the ECG machine needs to run at:
A any rate, provided it is slow enough
B 55 mm/sec
C 45 mm/sec
D 25 mm/sec

4 The calibration of the ECG machine needs to be set at:
A 1 mV represents 5 mm vertically
B 1 mV represents 10 mm vertically
C 1 mV represents 1 mm vertically
D 1 V represents 10 mm vertically

5 When an ECG has been recorded, you should also document on the reading:

A when the patient last ate or drank

B whether the patient consented to the ECG

C the presence of symptoms at the time of the recording, such as chest pain

D how many electrodes were used

27 Performing cardiopulmonary resuscitation

1 When performing CPR, it is important to:

A follow the standardised algorithm

B minimise any pauses in compressions

C call for help as soon as possible

D all of the above

2 Reversible causes of arrest to consider include:

A cardiac tamponade

B hypovolaemia

C hypoxia

D all of the above

3 Chest compressions on an adult patient should be at a rate of:

A that which is clinically indicated, varying with patient size

B 100 to 120 compressions / min

C 60 to 80 compressions / min

D 80 to 100 compressions / min

4 The ratio of breaths to compressions in an adult patient should be:

A 15 breaths to 1 compression

B 1 breath to 15 compressions

C 30 breaths to 2 compressions

D 2 breaths to 30 compressions

5 Shockable rhythms, which require defibrillation, include:

A atrial tachycardia and atrial fibrillation

B ventricular tachycardia and ventricular fibrillation

C asystole and pulseless electrical activity

D ventricular asystole

28 Inserting a nasogastric tube

1 A nasogastric tube is:

A a thin wire inserted into the patient's stomach in a surgical procedure

B a tube attached to a valve for actively suctioning a patient's stomach

C a plastic tube inserted into a patient's stomach via their nostril

D a tube which bypasses a patient's stomach

2 A Ryle's tube is:

A another name for any nasogastric tube

B a large-bore tube

C a small-bore tube

D another name for a fine-bore tube

3 A Ryle's tube may be used for:

A feeding the patient

B decompressing an obstruction

C giving a patient fluids

D creating an obstruction

4 Nasogastric tubes should not be inserted if:

A there is no clinical indication

B there is significant facial trauma

C there are signs of a basal skull fracture

D all of the above

5 Prior to using a nasogastric tube for feeding:

A ask the patient if it feels comfortable

B order a chest X-ray

C confirm that the tip of the tube is in the correct location in the patient's stomach by seeing this on an X-ray

D confirm whether there are any other considerations and if it should be used immediately, especially if the patient is emaciated

29 Performing a digital rectal examination

1 A digital rectal examination may also be commonly referred to as a:

A BPE, for 'back passage examination'

B RE, for 'rectal examination'

C PA, for *per anus*

D PR, for *per rectum*

2 Prior to beginning the examination, you must:

A warn the patient that the examination will be painful

B offer the patient a chaperone

C advise the patient to empty their bladder

D ensure that the patient is lying supine

3 A digital rectal exam is generally considered part of a complete:

A cardiovascular examination

B neurology examination

C respiratory examination

D abdominal examination

4 A digital rectal examination may be most useful in the investigation of:

A constipation

B diabetes

C renal cell carcinoma

D pregnancy

5 After performing a digital rectal examination, you should document:

A if a chaperone was present

B the anal tone

C masses felt on palpation

D all of the above

30 Performing urinalysis

1 Urinalysis may be useful in investigating:

A pregnancy

B diabetes

C renal cell carcinoma

D all of the above

2 If the coloured pads on the urinalysis test strip indicate a presence of nitrites and leukocytes, it may most commonly indicate the presence of:
A diabetes
B urinary tract infection
C pregnancy
D obstructive jaundice

3 It is preferable to test a midstream urine (MSU) sample as:
A this sample is the most easy to obtain and requires no instructions to the patient
B this sample has less contamination
C this sample is difficult to obtain
D this sample has good conditions for sampling genital bacterial growth

4 Prior to performing urinalysis:
A ensure you have access to a timing device
B check the expiry date on the test strips
C correctly identify the patient
D all of the above

5 If a urinary tract infection is suspected, the MSU can also be sent for:
A chemistry and haematology
B biology and histology
C culture and sensitivity
D chemistry and histology

31 Inserting a bladder catheter

1 A bladder catheter is inserted through the:
A urethra
B ureter
C bladder
D abdomen

2 Bladder catheters can be used for:
A fluid balance monitoring in acutely unwell patients
B urinary retention
C bladder irrigation after bladder surgery
D all of the above

3 If you are having trouble inserting a bladder catheter:
A force it through any resistance felt
B try again but wait several hours, irrespective of how urgent the catheter is
C ask for senior help
D ask the patient to insert it

4 To insert the bladder catheter, you should use:
A non-sterile gloves and some care
B the aseptic non-touch technique
C force
D no local anaesthetic

5 After inserting a catheter, you should document:
A the reason for its insertion
B the residual volume drained
C details of the catheter used
D all of the above

32 Performing otoscopy

1 Otoscopy may performed to investigate:
A hearing loss
B tinnitus

C facial weakness
D all of the above

2 Some medications can cause hearing loss, including:
A antibiotics such as penicillin
B salicylates such as aspirin
C steroids such as hydrocortisone
D anti-depressants such as sertraline

3 A normal ear drum is most commonly:
A translucent and pink-grey in colour
B opaque and cream in colour
C solid and orange in colour
D translucent and blue in colour

4 When performing otoscopy in a child, pull their ear:
A vertically downwards
B vertically upwards
C diagonally outwards
D horizontally backwards

5 Prior to performing otoscopy:
A fully identify the patient
B inspect the outer ear
C place on a new disposal cap over the otoscope earpiece
D all of the above

33 Performing ophthalmoscopy

1 Ophthalmoscopy should be included as a part of a full and complete:
A cardiovascular exam
B neurological exam
C respiratory exam
D abdominal exam

2 Prior to performing ophthalmoscopy, it may be necessary to:
A sedate the patient
B dilate the patient's pupil with a nicotinic agent
C dilate the patient's pupil with an anti-muscarinic agent
D dilate the patient's pupil with adrenaline

3 An important side effect of 0.5% tropicamide is:
A itching
B acute angle-closure glaucoma
C dizziness
D wide-angle lens obstruction

4 When performing ophthalmoscopy:
A ensure you check for the red reflex
B ensure you check for the black reflex
C ensure you check for hyperacusis
D ensure you check for the lateral reflex

5 Another name for ophthalmoscopy is:
A optoscopy
B otoscopy
C fundoscopy
D visioscopy

34 Confirming and certifying death

1 Some deaths must be referred to coroner, including those due to:
A unknown causes
B recent medical procedures
C drugs
D all of the above

2 A Medical Certificate of the Cause of Death (MCCD) can only be issued by a doctor who had seen the patient in the last:

A 7 days

B 14 days

C 1 month

D 3 months

3 On the MCCD, Section 1a) refers to:

A general conditions the patient suffered from

B any conditions present at the time of death

C the specific condition which caused the death

D any factors which may have contributed to the death

4 In confirming death clinically, you should:

A check for an absence of response to pain

B check for an absence of circulation

C check for an absence of respiration

D all of the above

5 When confirming death, it is advisable to also check for:

A false teeth

B a hip replacement

C a pacemaker

D previous surgery

Multiple choice answers

1 Overview of practical procedures

1 A

Practical procedures are required to deliver quality patient care. Proficiency in many practical procedures is currently a regulated recommendation by the General Medical Council.

2 D

Practical procedures, such as venepuncture, occur every day, many times per day, in most clinical environments. These procedures can be used to help diagnose conditions, and to monitor their treatment, such as by looking at the rise and fall of inflammatory markers in blood to indicate the possible presence of infection, and the effects of antibiotics.

3 C

Always seek senior help with performing procedures – especially in instances where you do not feel confident in performing it, you have not performed it before or you feel it may be more complicated than you feel capable of managing.

4 B

Depending upon the local protocols of each Healthcare Trust, some nursing staff may be able to perform some practical procedures, such as venepuncture. This varies widely, so ensure that you are familiar with that which is permitted in each area you work in.

5 D

It is the medical professional's responsibility to ensure that no harm is done to the patient, as per the Hippocratic Oath. Local policies must be adhered to, as must current 'best practice', to ensure that optimal patient care is delivered each time.

2 Non-technical skills

1 D

Communication includes many different components, and in order to communicate most effectively, it may be appropriate to use many different forms to convey meaning. Written words, actions and spoken words are all important parts of communication.

2 C

Communicating in areas where you may be overheard is not good practice, but if it is unavoidable, ensure the patient's confidentiality is maximised. It is not good practice to use family members as translators, as in some cases, the patient may not receive impartial information or may not feel able to convey their wishes openly. Effective communication is maximised by appropriate levels of eye contact and a posture that is suitably attentive and open.

3 B

Task management involves prioritising activities in the order of importance. Other factors such as difficulty,

duration, cost or ease should not be the primary dictator of when tasks are done – they should be done in the order of importance.

4 D

Situation awareness involves many aspects. It involves modifying a workspace to gain maximum information, as well as asking questions to maximise understanding of this information. It involves observing, interpreting and comprehending this information, as well as anticipating what may occur.

5 B

Teamwork involves multiple aspects, all of which are facilitated by good communication skills. It involves allocating roles based upon each member's capabilities and limitations, after discussing and recognising these. These roles need to be respected and accepted by the team members, and for all members to then work in co-operation.

3 Waste, sharps disposal and injuries

1 D

Local policies may vary in each Healthcare Trust; however, generally bins for clinical waste are yellow and clearly marked.

2 B

Ensure that waste is disposed of in the correct bins. Pay particular care in respecting patient confidentiality, and ensuring that any confidential waste containing patient information is disposed of in confidential waste bins.

3 D

Never re-sheathe a needle, and always use the attached needle-safe units if one is present. These help minimise the risk of an injury by protecting you from the needle. Sharps must always be disposed of in a sharps bin, ideally in a portable one that you can have with you to facilitate immediate disposal after use.

4 C

Sharps injuries must be dealt with immediately, by encouraging bleeding under running water, and washing it with soap. Occupational Health must be contacted immediately, and they generally will help with future steps such as patient testing for possible relevant illnesses such as hepatitis and HIV.

5 B

Soiled incontinence products should be disposed of in yellow clinical waste bins, along with any contaminated products such as dressings, aprons, and gloves. Food wrappers should be disposed of in domestic waste bins, while anything with patient details on it should be disposed of in a confidential waste bin.

4 Identifying a patient

1 D

Patient identification is of utmost importance, and thus they must be identified at the start of each encounter, and with multiple data points. They must also be wearing a wristband if they are in hospital, which has not been tampered with.

2 B

Incorrect identification of a patient is a 'never event', as decreed by the Department of Health, and must not happen. If it does, there are harsh penalties for the Healthcare Trust involved, even if there is minimal harm to the patient as an outcome.

3 B

It is not advisable for you to ask 'Are you …?' as this breaches the other patient's confidentiality, whilst potentially also confusing the patient you are addressing. Even if you have evidence such as a name board, or a member of staff has already told you the patient's name, you must always fully identify them at the start of a clinical encounter.

4 A

Studies have indicated that half of all hospital errors were preventable, which led to the 5 Patient Safety Rights being formalised.

5 D

The 5 Patient Safety Rights are (1) ensuring the right patient (2) is given the right treatment (3) in the right dose (4) through the right route (5) at the right time. As a medical professional, it is your duty to help maintain these rights.

5 Consent, capacity and documentation

1 C

Consent is only valid if it is given voluntarily, and thus without coercion, and if it is given when the patient has capacity.

2 B

A patient must be able to communicate their decision, but this may be by forms other than talking in some cases. Whilst a patient with capacity may refuse treatment, this is not an aspect of assessing capacity. Capacity is required for consenting, whilst the inverse does not hold true.

3 B

Many cases are confusing and difficult to determine, and senior help should be sought in cases where the clinician is unsure. Other experts are able to decide capacity. Capacity is an entity which may be present or absent, but can change with the patient's condition.

4 A

A patient has the right to withdraw their consent, if they have capacity at the time when they wish to do this. Consent is required for all interventions, from the small and non-invasive, to the large and invasive.

5 C

In some instances, consent may be spoken, such as a patient verbally agreeing to a blood sample being taken from their arm. In some cases, such as surgery, it must be informed, documented and written formally. In some cases it may be implied, such as a patient extending their arm for a blood pressure cuff to be attached, so that their vital signs can be measured.

6 Hand hygiene and personal protective equipment

1 D

To thoroughly wash the hands, there are six basic motions that should be used to ensure the maximum chance of hand cleanliness. This should occur at five different moments in a clinical interaction – before talking to the patient, before a task, after the risk of bodily fluid contact, after patient contact and after contact with the patient's surroundings.

2 B

PPE is commonly used to represent 'personal protective equipment'. This includes, but is not limited to, gloves, masks, caps, booties, aprons and goggles.

3 D

Hands should be cleaned both before and after the use of gloves, as studies have indicated that microbes can 'flourish' in the environment inside the glove, and thus hands are contaminated when the gloves are removed

4 B

Alcoholic rubs are a useful addition to hand hygiene, as they are easy to use. They are used frequently in hospitals, and are effective for removing many types of bacteria. They are not effective against some bacteria, such as *C. difficile*, and therefore other types of hand hygiene such as handwashing with an antibacterial agent and water are still required.

5 C

Hand hygiene is one of the most important methods for minimising disease transmission, as hands are one of the most common vectors for disease transmission. Adequate cleaning helps break the transmission cycle.

7 Scrubbing in

1 C

Scrubbing in may be known by various terms, but generally 'scrubbing up' or 'surgical scrubbing' are common. It refers to a thorough cleaning process, and the donning of sterile personal protective equipment in preparation for some invasive procedures or theatre.

2 A

Iodine-based solutions are brownish in colour, while the chlorhexidine-based solutions are pinkish in colour. These two solutions are most commonly used for scrubbing in, as soap and gels are not sufficiently antibacterial.

3 C

If you accidentally touch a non-sterile surface, you have de-sterilised yourself before you begin the procedure, and you are placing the patient at a greater risk of infection. Start the scrubbing-in process again, after letting a colleague know what has happened, so that they are aware of the possibility of a slight delay.

4 D

Once you have scrubbed in, move carefully around and touch nothing so that you do not de-sterilise yourself. Non-sterile items such as your cap, mask and shoes cannot be touched as these will de-sterilise you – if they require adjustment, ask a (non-scrubbed-in) colleague to assist you.

5 A

Ensure you have collected all of the correct equipment, and you have donned the appropriate PPE prior to starting scrubbing in. When you start, take your time, and take care. If you de-sterilise yourself and need to start again, do not worry. It is better to begin again than to introduce an infection to the patient.

8 Asepsis

1 A

ANTT aims to minimise the risk of infectious contamination. It is used as a pre-procedure prior to many invasive procedures, and does not replace other steps such as handwashing.

2 D

All invasive procedures should be approached with ANTT, in order to minimise the risk of contamination.

3 B

Key sites are very important to identify and recognise. They are areas where infection can easily be introduced into the body during a procedure, and thus particular care must be taken to not touch them. Key sites include wounds, puncture sites and insertion sites for a catheter or a cannula.

4 A

A key part is very important to identify, as it can easily introduce infection into the patient if it is contaminated. The concept of key parts and key sites is very important, as key parts must only come into contact with key sites, and both must remain uncontaminated.

5 D

All of the above pieces are key parts, they must remain uncontaminated and only these parts can touch key sites.

9 Measuring vital signs

1 A

Respiratory rate is routinely measured in patients as a vital sign, and it is a good clinical indicator of if a patient is deteriorating. Other parameters may only be measured if clinically indicated. Appetite and mood may be recorded for patients, for example if they are depressed. Weight may be measured in some instances, for example if they are being treated for fluid overload.

2 D

Vital signs measurements can be viewed as one-off absolute values, and as markers of a state at a particular time, but also as parts of clinical trends, showing possibly a decline or improvement in physiology.

3 C

Oxygen saturation is commonly measured with a probe clipped onto the patient's finger, or clipped onto the patient's

ear. Remember to record the inspired oxygen level for the oxygen saturation level to be read in a clinically relevant context.

4 D

Temperature can be measured in many ways – including rectally, sublingually or tympanically – with the latter being the most common method.

5 A

Generally, the heart rate is measured at a peripheral pulse such as the radial artery.

10 Writing a safe prescription

1 B

OD represents *omne in die*, or once a day. BD represents *bis in die*, or twice a day. TDS represents *ter die sumendum*, or three times a day. PRN represents *pro re nata*, or as needed/as required. QDS represents *quarter die sumendus*, or four times a day. ON represents *omne nocte*, or every night; and PR represents *per rectum*, or via the rectum.

2 D

Prescriptions should name medications generically, be clear, legible, and written in pen. They should also have the prescriber's bleep number and signature, amongst other information, included.

3 A

Patients who are overloaded, or who have a compromised cardiovascular system or various other comorbidities, may require slower IV fluids. This rule is not absolute, and it varies with clinical situations.

4 C

Oxygen is a drug, and therefore it must be prescribed by a doctor. The prescription should indicate the timeframe over which it is to be administered, including if this is continuous or intermittently according to saturations. Oxygen saturations vary with some conditions – for instance, it is appropriate to aim for 88–92% in patients with chronic pulmonary obstructive disorder, whilst patients without such lung pathologies should have target saturations of 94–98%.

5 C

Generally, 'units' and 'micro' should be written in full, to avoid errors, although this may differ with hospital policies. Commonly PRN is used widely, standing for *pro re nata*, or as required. Prescriptions must always be written in pen.

11 Performing venepuncture

1 C

Gentle palpation should be used to select veins for venepuncture – it helps determine a vein of sufficient volume for the sample to be successfully taken. The palpation should be gentle, as if it is too firm, the veins will collapse under the pressure.

2 D

Many different anatomical areas may be used for venepuncture – commonly the antecubital fossa is used. A-V fistulae and regions of cellulitis and phlebitis should be avoided if possible.

3 C

This angle of insertion and bevel orientation make full use of the surface area of the needle bevel exposed to the vein without piercing the posterior wall.

4 D

Venepuncture is useful for monitoring levels of physiological parameters, and of medications, in the blood.

5 D

You do not fill the vials in a random order when collecting blood samples. Some vials contain additives which may act as contaminants for other vials, if they are filled before them. This varies with local Healthcare Trust protocols.

12 Taking blood cultures

1 C

If a patient has consented, there is an indication and the relevant equipment is available, blood cultures can be taken. An ECG may be useful for other clinical information, but it is not needed prior to blood cultures being taken.

2 C

Anaerobic organisms exist when no oxygen is present. Blood cultures are taken to look at the presence of bacteria in the blood, not to indicate drug levels or therapy effects.

3 B

Aerobic samples should be taken first, and other blood samples should be collected after the blood culture samples have been collected.

4 A

Blood cultures are processed in the Microbiology Department. Haematology processes requests such as blood films, whilst Chemistry and Biochemistry process requests to do with parameters such as liver function. These vary according to local hospital protocols.

5 D

Blood cultures may be taken for various clinically indicated reasons, including elevated temperature and septic signs.

13 Inserting a cannula in a peripheral vein

1 D

The cannula provides intravenous access, so it may be used whenever direct administration into the vein is required.

2 B

The area must be thoroughly cleaned prior to insertion of the cannula, with chlorhexidine wipes the preferred method. Cannulation is a mini surgical procedure, and thus must be performed with ANTT.

3 B

A small window at the back of the cannula shows blood when it is first inserted into the vein. Secondary flashback appears when it is advanced further, and this is seen in the tube of the cannula itself.

4 A

Blood samples can only be taken the first time a cannula is inserted. Even if the end of the cannula or its bung are cleaned, later samples cannot be taken. The correct equipment must be used when the samples are taken.

5 D

Veins should be gently palpated to ensure that they are of sufficient volume for the cannula. As the cannula remains *in situ*, and as the introducing needle is straight, it is preferable to select a straight vein, as this minimises the risk of failure.

14 Measuring blood glucose

1 B

Blood glucose measurements are useful and quick to obtain, but at times they may be inaccurate. They are used frequently. They should therefore be checked in the laboratory, by collecting a sample by venepuncture and sending this off to the laboratory for processing.

2 C

The lancet contains a small needle, which is spring loaded to prick the patient's finger. After use, this must be disposed of in a clinical sharps bin.

3 D

The patient may have a preferred finger for testing; however, it is usually least painful to use the pulp on the side of the medial two digits on their non-dominant hand. (Remember that the body is described in the anatomical position – palms forward, and thus thumbs pointing out. Therefore, the medial two digits are the two digits closest to the anatomical mid-line, the 'pinky' and the 'ring finger'.)

4 D

Confusion, tremor and palpitations may all be present in a patient with hypoglycaemia, and therefore a blood glucose measurement may be indicated.

5 D

Reagent strips have an expiry date that must be checked prior to use. As with any clinical interaction, the patient needs to be fully identified. The lancet used to obtain the sample must be disposed of in a clinical sharps bin, thus it is preferable to locate one of these prior to commencing.

15 Suturing

1 C

Both Monocryl and Vicryl are absorbable sutures, whilst Prolene is non-absorbable. Steri-strips are not sutures, but are external adhesive strips to assist in wound closure.

2 D

Sutures, glue, staples and steri-strips are all commonly used methods for closing wounds. Which is used depends upon the clinical indication, contra-indications and other parameters.

3 D

The patient needs to be correctly identified prior to any intervention. The tetanus status and any neurovascular deficit must also be established prior to wound closure.

4 C

The timeframe is approximate, as it varies according to many parameters, for example wound depth, skin integrity and comorbidities such as diabetes.

5 B

Slightly everting the skin enables optimal healing. If the edges are inverted, level or overlapping, there may be slower wound healing, increased infection risk or a poorer cosmetic outcome.

16 Administering intravenous infusions

1 B

If a cannula is *in situ*, there are no signs of infection and the cannula has been in for an acceptable timeframe according to local policies, it may be used for the administration of fluids. Prior to use, it must be flushed, to ensure that it is patent and not clotted. It does not need to be removed or replaced if it is infection free and functional. It must also be flushed after use.

2 C

Gelofusin® and blood should be given via colloid giving sets. Saline can be given using a crystalloid giving set.

3 B

Prior to using a giving set, it needs to be primed. This is done by attaching sterile saline and letting it flow through the entire length of the tube, prior to connecting the fluid that requires administration. This is done to remove air from the line, reducing the risk of air embolism.

4 C

If a steady delivery rate is required, or the infusion must be delivered over a specific timeframe, a pump can be used. These provide a more controlled and more predictable delivery of the fluids.

5 D

Prior to connection, the end of the cannula must be wiped with a chlorhexidine wipe. Key sites and key parts should never be touched. The roller should not be opened until the line has been connected to the cannula, or fluid will run out over the floor and the patient.

17 Administrating intravenous infusions of blood and blood products

1 C

A sample of blood must be specifically tested for the group in order to determine the patient's blood group. Verbal confirmation from a patient or relative is insufficient, and blood cultures are not for determining blood groups.

2 D

Blood group O is referred to as a universal donor, as all main blood types can receive this blood. Other blood types may be incompatible, due to the antibodies they possess.

3 A

Some patients may refuse blood or its products for religious reasons. A patient cannot request blood if it is not clinically indicated. A patient cannot refuse blood if they do not have capacity, and they should be treated in their best interests.

4 A

All details should be checked by yourself, and again with a colleague, upon receipt of the blood and again at the patient's bedside prior to administering the transfusion.

5 B

The patient must have their vital signs monitored frequently during a transfusion, to watch for signs of reactions. The patient is permitted to move as is clinically appropriate and does not interfere with their monitoring – they do not need to remain absolutely still, and they are able to eat and drink if appropriate.

18 Administering parenteral medications

1 C

When drawing up medications, a fine-gauge needle or a filter/drawing-up needle should be used, in order to remove any particles or shards of glass prior to injection. Only some medications are available in pre-packaged kits.

2 A

Medications must be thoroughly mixed prior to administering them, to ensure that the correct dose is given – this is particularly important with infusions such as an insulin sliding scale.

3 B

Medication doses may vary with routes of administration, due to the differences that occur with metabolism and absorption. It is best to check this, and to also check the dose required with other conditions – such as, for example, renal or liver impairment, and pregnancy.

4 D

Prior to administering medications, ensure that the patient consents to receiving it, and is not allergic to it. Ensure that the medication is not past its expiry date. All of these aspects, and several others, should be checked prior to administration of the medication.

5 A

Some medications will require additional monitoring to be implemented. Ensure that you do this yourself, as best practice – or ensure that it is clearly handed over to the appropriate healthcare practitioner so that it is commenced in a clinically appropriate timeframe. For example, an insulin sliding scale will require blood glucose level monitoring. Additional unused medication cannot be replaced into its original vials, and must be disposed of if no longer needed.

19 Administering injections

1 A

Aspirate, by pulling back on the syringe plunger slightly, to ensure that you are not in a blood vessel, prior to giving an injection. Keep the needle still, and inject at a steady rate, slowly but as clinically indicated. Repeated injections may require different sites, but this should be determined prior to inserting the needle.

2 D

If a patient is refusing the injection, and they have capacity, then this refusal must be adhered to. Speak to a senior, or find other possible routes of administration if this is the case. If a patient has had a previous anaphylactic reaction to a medication, this is a contra-indication against giving it. Avoid injecting into areas of infection if possible.

3 C

Generally, a needle of a smaller gauge should be used to administer injections intradermally, and a larger gauge needle for administering injections intramuscularly.

4 B

Intradermal injections provide very localised administration of a medication. For systemic delivery, intramuscular or subcutaneous injections are needed, and intramuscular injections are faster acting than subcutaneous injections.

5 C

Generally, intramuscular injections are the most painful type of injection, as the muscle into which the medication is placed has little ability to accommodate it. By comparison, intradermal, intravenous and subcutaneous regions are generally less painful, as they are more able to accommodate the additional fluid.

20 Measuring arterial blood gas

1 C

An artery needs to be sampled, as it is an arterial blood gas (ABG) measurement. The ulnar artery is assessed for patency, as the radial artery is the preferred source, due to its anatomical location and dimensions.

2 B

The wrist should be dorsiflexed. This enables maximum exposure to the radial artery. Patients should be positioned to enable maximum comfort – generally sitting with their arm supported.

3 A

A modified Allen test should be performed to ensure that there is an adequate collateral circulation, prior to sampling the radial artery.

4 D

Air bubbles and clots can lead to false readings. Air bubbles must be expelled prior to analysis. Agitation with the heparin in the sample minimises the risk of clots. The results cannot be read without being put into context, thus the patient's oxygen therapy levels should be recorded also.

5 B

Haemoglobin (Hb) is usually measured on an ABG, although this may vary with different settings and different analysers.

21 Administering oxygen therapy

1 B

Oxygen therapy is used for a large number of patients, as hypoxaemia is present in many disease states. It is frequently used in emergency settings. Capacity and patient demands with regards to oxygen are the same as with any other medications – a patient without capacity may be treated with oxygen if there are clinical indications and it is in the patient's best interests. A patient requesting oxygen would ordinarily not be treated with it, unless there was a clinical indication. A sleepy patient may be treated with oxygen therapy if clinically indicated.

2 B

The oxygen saturations for a healthy adult are 94–98%, and these should be prescribed on the medication chart when the oxygen is prescribed. Target saturations of 88–92% are for an adult at risk of hypercapnic respiratory failure.

3 D

The highest percentage of inspired oxygen, at over 80%, is delivered by a non-rebreathe mask. Ensure that you fill the reservoir bag with oxygen prior to putting the mask on the patient.

4 C

A high oxygen requirement is a sign of illness severity. It should prompt frequent monitoring, and additional measures such as an ABG and input from a senior.

5 D

Oxygen is a medication and therefore must be prescribed on the patient's medication card. It should be reduced as tolerated by the patient, after consideration of the clinical picture.

22 Using inhalers and nebulisers

1 D

Inhalers and nebulisers are both used to deliver medications to the lungs, and thus these medications must be prescribed on the patient's medication card. They require different amounts of co-ordination to deliver the medications, with nebulisers requiring less than inhalers.

2 B

If a patient is having difficulty using an inhaler, it may be appropriate to consider attaching it to a spacer. You should also check their technique, as this may be the cause of the difficulties.

3 C

Some patients do not feel comfortable with the mask used for nebulised medications. If this is the case, and the patient definitely requires nebulised medications, consider using the handheld mouthpiece device instead as this may be more comfortable for them. It is not suitable to step down the treatment to an inhaler, or to step it up to intubation, if these are not clinically indicated.

4 D

Inhalers are commonly used in the treatment of respiratory conditions. In conditions such as asthma, they may be part of a step-wise program that is stepped up or stepped down to provide adequate symptom control. They can contain more than one medication in a single inhaler.

5 B

A nebuliser medication chamber requires approximately 4–10 ml of medication.

23 Assessing respiratory function

1 A

Peak flow meters measure a person's maximum rate of airflow during a sudden forced expiration starting from full inspiration. The other parameters can be measured by spirometry.

2 C

Total lung capacity cannot be measured by spirometry or by a peak flow meter; it must be measured by other techniques such as plethysmography. A nebuliser is used for the delivery of medications.

3 D

As with any clinical interaction, the patient must be fully identified. The peak flow meter needs to be zeroed to enable accurate readings to be taken, and a single-use disposal mouthpiece must be applied prior to use.

4 B

Peak flow readings are useful in conditions such as asthma. Conditions such as flu tend to be more short-lived, whilst conditions such as lung cancer have decreased variability, and thus peak flow readings are not generally as useful.

5 D

Peak flow readings vary with parameters such as age, gender and height.

24 Using airway manoeuvres and simple adjuncts

1 C

The three simple airway manoeuvres are the head tilt, chin lift and jaw thrust.

2 D

A nasopharyngeal airway and an oropharyngeal airway are both simple airway adjuncts which a junior medical professional is expected to be able to use. An LMA is a more specialised type of airway adjunct.

3 D

Nasopharyngeal airways should not generally be used if there is any clinical indication of a base-of-skull fracture. As with any clinical decision, the risks and benefits need to be weighed against each other, and the appropriate decision made after consideration of these facts.

4 B

To size an oropharyngeal airway, measure from the incisor to the angle of the jaw. There are various different sizes of airways available, and thus this must be correctly measured prior to insertion.

5 B

Suction should only be used under direct vision – thus, in areas which can be seen clearly. It may be used in patients of various ages, if clinically indicated.

25 Ventilating with a bag valve mask device

1 B

Bag valve mask devices are often used with airway adjuncts. They can be used in patients of different ages, if clinically indicated. They are used in hypoventilating patients, not hyperventilating patients, and should be used by two people, not only with one hand.

2 D

Bag valve mask devices are generally found on the resuscitation trolleys for use during cardiac arrests. This may vary with local Healthcare Trust policies, and they may also be found in other areas.

3 B

When applying the mask to the patient's face, hold your thumb and index finger in the shape of a 'C' on each side of the mask. This facilitates creating a good seal around the patient's face and the edge of the mask.

4 B

Squeezing the bag of the bag valve mask device delivers oxygen or air to the patient, depending on what is attached to the device. The device is often used in theatres but is not used to induce the patient with general anaesthetic.

5 B

Capnography produces a tracing which rises and falls with each breath, according to the levels of carbon dioxide being exhaled. Spirometry is for measuring aspects of lung function. A stethoscope may be helpful in clinically determining ventilation, by listening to the chest for breath sounds; however, capnography provides a more reliable objective method for assessing ventilation.

26 Recording a 12-lead electrocardiogram

1 B

To obtain a 12-lead electrocardiogram, six chest leads and four limb leads are required.

2 C

In an ECG, a positive deflection in the ECG waveform reflects depolarisation of that region of cardiac muscle flowing towards the electrode.

3 D

The paper in the ECG machine needs to be set at a standard rate, of 25 mm/sec. This must be checked prior to recording the ECG, as if it is recorded at the incorrect speed, the ECG is inaccurate.

4 B

The calibration of the ECG machine needs to be set such that 1 mV represents 10 mm vertically. If the machine is incorrectly calibrated, the ECG is inaccurate.

5 C

When an ECG has been recorded, you should also document on the reading the presence of symptoms at the time of the recording, such as chest pain. These help to place readings into clinical context. No investigation should be performed without a patient's consent; however, this does not need to be formally documented on the ECG reading. In a standard 12-lead ECG, 10 electrodes are used.

27 Performing cardiopulmonary resuscitation

1 D

When performing CPR, it is important to follow the standardised algorithm. It is important to minimise any pauses in compressions for activities such as rhythm checks, and it is vital to call for help or put out an arrest call as soon as possible.

2 D

There are many reversible causes to be considered in an arrest – these include hypoxia, hypovolaemia, hypothermia, metabolic derangement, tension pneumothorax, cardiac tamponade, toxins and thrombi.

3 B

Chest compressions on an adult patient should be at a rate of 100 to 120 compressions/min, at a depth of 5 to 6 cm.

4 D

The ratio of breaths to compressions in an adult patient should be 2 breaths to every 30 compressions.

5 B

Shockable rhythms, which require defibrillation, include ventricular tachycardia and ventricular fibrillation.

28 Inserting a nasogastric tube

1 C

A nasogastric tube is a plastic tube which is inserted into a patient's stomach via their nostril. It is not a wire, although some thin tubes may have a guide wire inside of the tube, which must be removed prior to usage. It is not for active suctioning a patient's stomach, although it can help in decompressing it if there is an obstruction. The tip of a nasogastric tube should sit in the patient's stomach – it should not bypass it.

2 B

A Ryle's tube is of a larger bore, and thus a larger diameter, than some other types of nasogastric tubes.

3 B

A Ryle's tube is useful for removing contents from a patient's stomach. It is therefore useful for patients who are in obstruction. Therefore, when it is inserted, it should have a drainage bag attached to it, to store the contents that are removed from the patient. Fine-bore nasogastric tubes should be used for feeding.

4 D

Nasogastric tubes should not be inserted if there is no indication that warrants one clinically. They should also not be inserted if there are signs of trauma, or signs of basal skull fractures, such as sub-orbital bruising (Panda eyes) or retro-auricular bruising (Battel's sign).

5 C

Correct siting of the nasogastric tube needs to be verified radiologically prior to it being used for feeding. A chest X-ray not only must be requested, but also must be reviewed and the NG tube's location confirmed prior to use.

29 Performing a digital rectal examination

1 D

A digital rectal examination may commonly be referred to as a PR, as an abbreviation of *per rectum*.

2 B

Prior to beginning a digital rectal examination, you must offer the patient a chaperone – this is for their safety and comfort, as well as your own. Generally, the examination should not hurt – thus, the patient should be advised that the examination may be uncomfortable, but should not be painful. The patient does not need to empty their bladder prior to examination, and they should be examined lying in the lateral position.

3 D

A digital rectal exam is generally considered part of a complete abdominal examination. It may be indicated in other examinations, such as if a neurology examination is being performed for a patient with suspected cauda equine or spinal cord compression, or as clinically indicated.

4 A

Any alteration in bowel habit, such as constipation or diarrhoea, should prompt a digital rectal examination to be performed.

5 D

After performing a digital rectal examination, you must fully document the examination and its findings. This includes the presence of a chaperone, and, if one is not present, the offer and declining of one should be recorded in the patient notes. On examination, inspection and palpation findings should be recorded, as should other parameters such as anal tone.

30 Performing urinalysis

1 D

Urinalysis is a simple test used frequently in clinical practice. It can be used in the investigation of many various conditions such as pregnancy and diabetes, and pathologies such as renal cell carcinoma and glomerulonephritis.

2 B

Most commonly, the presence of nitrites and leukocytes may indicate the presence of a urinary tract infection.

3 B

It is preferable to test an MSU as this sample generally has less contamination from bacterial commensals that are normally present on the skin of the genitals. The sample is not too difficult to obtain, but it does require clear instructions to the patient about which part of the stream to collect, and the importance of retracting the foreskin or parting the labia.

4 D

As with any clinical encounter, the patient needs to be correctly identified. The test strips have expiry dates on them, which must be checked prior to use. In order to read these test strips accurately, the time that lapsed since the exposure to the urine must be timed, as different sections of the strip react at different times and need to therefore be read at different precise time intervals.

5 C

An MSU can be sent for culture and sensitivity, if a urinary tract infection is suspected. This enables the pathogens to be cultured and grown, and their sensitivities to different antibiotics to be determined.

31   Inserting a bladder catheter

1 A

A bladder catheter is inserted via the urethra, into the bladder where it terminates, acting to drain the bladder contents. A supra-pubic catheter may be inserted into the bladder through the abdominal wall.

2 D

Bladder catheters may be inserted for a range of reasons, including but not limited to monitoring fluid balance in an acutely unwell patient, urinary retention and post-operative bladder irrigation, and for surgical procedures.

3 C

Ask for senior help, rather than forcing a catheter in or delaying its insertion, if you are having trouble inserting it. Do not continue forcing it in, as you may create a false passage by damaging the urethra, causing further problems for the patient.

4 B

To insert the catheter, you should use sterile gloves and a strict aseptic non-touch technique. Local anaesthetic should be instilled in the urethra prior to insertion (provided that there are no contra-indications to it), to minimise discomfort for the patient.

5 D

After inserting the catheter, a significant amount of important information needs to be recorded in the patient's notes. This includes the indication, date, time, details of the catheter (usually available as a sticker from the catheter packaging), technique used, residual volume drained and any problems or complications encountered.

32   Performing otoscopy

1 D

Otoscopy may be performed to investigate symptoms of ear disease – these include hearing loss, vertigo, tinnitus, otorrhoea, otalgia and facial pain.

2 B

Medications can cause hearing loss. These can include loop diuretics such as furosemide, and salicylates such as aspirin.

3 A

A normal eardrum is almost translucent and appears pink-grey in colour. A very red ear drum may be a sign of otitis media.

4 D

In a child, pull the ear horizontally backwards, whereas in an adult, pull the ear upwards and backwards, to perform otoscopy.

5 D

As with any clinical interaction, fully identify the patient. Place a clean disposable cap over the otoscope earpiece prior to use, and the outer ear should be thoroughly inspected prior to inserting the otoscope.

33   Performing ophthalmoscopy

1 B

Ophthalmoscopy should be included as part of any complete neurological exam.

2 C

Prior to performing ophthalmoscopy, it may be necessary to dilate the patient's pupil with an anti-muscarinic agent. 0.5% tropicamide is commonly used for this purpose. As with any medication, it is important to check for allergies and contra-indications prior to administration.

3 B

Acute angle-closure glaucoma can develop as an important and serious side effect of the use of dilating drops such as 0.5% tropicamide. It is an emergency.

4 A

Ensure that you check for the red reflex, which involves shining the ophthalmoscope into the patient's eyes from an arm's-length distance. This should be done prior to closely approaching the patient, and it is done to check for the presence of conditions such as cataracts.

5 C

Ophthalmoscopy is also known as fundoscopy.

34   Confirming and certifying death

1 D

Various causes of death must be referred to a coroner; those include, but are not limited to, deaths from drugs, suicides or unknown causes. Deaths in less than 24 hours after admission to hospital or those due to recent medical procedures must also be referred.

2 B

An MCCD can only be issued by a doctor who had seen the patient in the last 14 days prior to their death.

3 C

On the MCCD, there are various sections. Section 1a) refers to the specific condition which caused the death. Sections 1b) and 1c) relate to any other diseases which may have contributed to the death, but not specifically caused it.

4 D

In confirming death, you must clinically verify that no response to pain, no circulation and no respiration are present in the patient.

5 C

When confirming death, it is advisable to also check for a pacemaker by palpating the subclavicular region on the patient. Certain pacemakers and implantable cardiac devices are inappropriate for cremation, and thus their presence must be noted and recorded.

Further reading and references

It is imperative to consult and adhere to the information provided by local Healthcare Trusts, and national and international advisory and regulatory bodies. Their resources are continuously updated and therefore should be checked frequently, to ensure that best current practices are adopted and maintained.

The following texts are highly recommended as general learning resources, and they have also been specifically consulted in the writing of this book. The resources listed under each chapter are specifically pertinent to that chapter, but they may also have been used in other areas of the book:

Blundell A, Harrison R, *OSCEs at a Glance*, 2nd edition, 2013, Wiley Blackwell, Oxford.

Borley NR, *Surgery at a Glance*, 5th edition, 2013, Wiley Blackwell, Oxford.

Carney, S. Gallen D, *The Foundation Programme at a Glance*, 2014, Wiley Blackwell, Oxford.

British Medical Association: www.bma.com

British Medical Journal: www.bmj.com

Davey P, *Medicine at a Glance,* 3rd edition, 2013, Wiley Blackwell, Oxford.

Faiz O, Moffat D, *Anatomy at a Glance*, 2nd edition, 2008, Wiley Blackwell, Oxford.

Gleadle J, *History and Examination at a Glance*, 3rd edition, 2012, Wiley Blackwell, Oxford.

Grace PA, Longmore M, Wilsonson I, Turmezei T, Cheung CK, *Oxford Handbook of Clinical Medicine*, 7th edition, 2008, Oxford University Press, Oxford.

National Health Service: www.nhs.uk

National Institute for Health and Care Excellence: www.nice.org.uk

Raine, T, McGinn K, Dawson J, Sanders S, Eccles S, *Oxford Handbook for the Foundation Programme*, 3rd edition, 2011, Oxford University Press, Oxford.

Ramrakha P, Moore K, Sam A, *Oxford Handbook of Acute Medicine*, 3rd edition, 2011, Oxford University Press, Oxford.

Stephenson M, Shur J, Black J, *How to Perform Clinical Procedures*, 2013, Wiley Blackwell, Oxford.

Thomas J, Monaghan T, *Oxford Handbook of Clinical Examination and Practical Skills*, 2010, Oxford University Press, Oxford.

Tomorrow's Doctors: http://www.gmc-uk.org/TomorrowsDoctors_2009.pdf_39260971.pdf

Chapter 1

British Medical Association: www.bma.org.uk

General Medical Council: www.gmc-uk.org

National Institute for Health and Care Excellence: www.nice.org.uk

Tomorrow's Doctors: www.gmc-uk.org/TomorrowsDoctors_2009.pdf_39260971.pdf

Chapter 2

Fletcher G, Flin R, McGeorge P, Glavin R, Maran N, Patey R. Anaesthetists' Non-Technical Skills (ANTS): Evaluation of a Behavioural Marker System. *Br. J. Anaesth.* (2003) 90 (5): 580–588.

Flin R, O'Connor P, Crichton M, *Safety at the Sharp End: A Guide to Non-Technical Skills*, 2008, Ashgate, Aldershot.

Chapter 3

National Health Service: www.nhs.uk

Chapter 4

Department of Health, Coding for Success, and Implementation of Coding for Success, 'never events': www.gov.uk/government/organisations/department-of-health

GS1, Healthcare Reference Book: www.gs1.org/docs/healthcare/case_studies/Case_study_UK_Coding_for_success.pdf

National Patient Safety Agency, Safer Practice Notice, Right Patient – Right Care: Improving Patient Safety through Better Manual and Technology-Based Systems for Identification and Matching of Patients with Care: www.nrls.npsa.nhs.uk www.npsa.nhs.uk

World Health Organization: http://www.who.int/patientsafety/education/curriculum/course11_handout.pdf

Chapter 5

Hope A, Savulsecu J, Hendrick J, *Medical Ethics and the Law,* 2nd edition, 2008, Elsevier, Oxford.

Mental Capacity Act 2005: www.legislation.gov.uk/ukpga/2005/9/part/1

Medical Defence Union: www.thedu.com

Medical Protection Society: www.medicalprotection.org

Scottish Law: www.scottishlaw.org.uk/journal/mar2001/sclubgilmar01.pdf

Chapter 6

Ayliffe GA, Babb JR, Quoraishi AH. A Test for 'Hygienic' Hand Disinfection. *J. Clin. Pathol.* (1978) 31: 923–928. doi:10.1136/jcp.31.10.923

Clean Your Hands Campaign: www.npsa.nhs.uk/cleanyourhands

Control of Substances Hazardous to Health (COSHH): www.hse.gov.uk

Sax H, Allegranzi B, Uçkay I, Larson E, Boyce J, Pittet D. 'My Five Moments for Hand Hygiene': A User-Centred Design Approach to Understand, Train, Monitor and Report Hand Hygiene. *J. Hosp. Infect.* (2007) 67: 9–21.

World Health Organization, *Hand Hygiene When and How Patient Safety Leaflet*, 2009, World Health Organization, Geneva.

Chapter 7

See resources listed above.

Chapter 8

Aseptic Non-Touch Technique: www.antt.org

Rowley S, Clare S, Macqueen S, Molyneux R. ANTT v2: An Updated Practice Framework for Aseptic Technique. *Brit. J. Nurs.* (2010) 19: S5–S11.

Chapter 9

Jahangir E, Blood Pressure Assessment, Medscape, http://emedicine.medscape.com/article/1948157-overview

Perloff D, Grim C, Flack J, Frohlich ED, Hill M, McDonald M. Human Blood Pressure Determination by Sphygmomanometry. *Circulation* (1993) 88 (5 Pt 1): 2460–2470.

Subbe C, Kruger M, Rutherford P, Gemmel L. Validation of a Modified Early Warning Score in Medical Admissions. *QJM* (2001) 94: 521–526.

Chapter 10

British Medical Association and the Royal Pharmaceutical Society of Great Britain, British National Formulary ('The BNF'), London (updated 6 monthly): www.bnf.org

National Institute for Health and Care Excellence: www.nice.org.uk

Nicholson T, Gunarathne A, Singer D, *Pocket Prescriber*, 2010, Hodder Education, Abington.

Chapter 11

Stephenson M, Shur J, Black J, *How to Perform Clinical Procedures*, 2013, John Wiley & Sons Ltd., Oxford.

Chapter 12

Patient.co.uk: www.patient.co.uk

Surviving Sepsis, The Sepsis Six: www.survivingsepsis.org, http://survivesepsis.org/the-sepsis-six

Chapter 13

Nagaratnam K, Torok E (IV Access Working Group), *VIP (Visual Infusion Phlebitis) Score*, n.d., Oxford Radcliff Hospitals NHS Trust, Oxford.

Chapter 15

Macafee D, Shah S, Singh S, *Suture Techniques for Staff and Students in Medicine and Nursing*, 2nd edition, Ethicon Products, Livingstone, Scotland.

Chapter 17

Taylor, C, Cohen H, Mold D, Jones H, *et al.*, Serious Hazards of Transfusion (SHOT) Steering Group, 2010: www.shotuk.org

UK Blood Transfusion and Tissue Transplantation Guidelines: www.transfusionguidelines.org.uk

Chapter 18

British Medical Association and the Royal Pharmaceutical Society of Great Britain, British National Formulary ('The BNF'), London (updated 6 monthly): www.bnf.org

Control of Substances Hazardous to Health (COSHH): www.hse.gov.uk

Chapter 20

British Thoracic Society: www.brit-thoracic.org.uk

Resuscitation Council, 5 Step Approach for Arterial Blood Gas Interpretation: www.resus.org.uk

Scottish Intercollegiate Guidelines Network: www.sign.ac.uk

World Health Organization, WHO Guidelines on Drawing Blood – Best Practices in Phlebotomy, Modified Allen Test: www.ncbi.nlm.nih.gov/books/NBK138652/

Chapter 21

Ward JPT, Ward J, Leach RM, *The Respiratory System at a Glance*, 3rd edition, 2010, John Wiley & Sons Ltd., Oxford.

Chapter 24

Leach R, *Critical Care Medicine at a Glance*, 2004, Wiley Blackwell, Oxford.

Chapter 26

ECGs – a Methodical Approach: www.patient.co.uk

Resuscitation Council: www.resus.org.uk

Chapter 27

Carney S, Gallen D, *The Foundation Programme at a Glance*, 2014, John Wiley & Sons Ltd., Oxford.

Resuscitation Council, Adult BLS Algorithm, ALS Algorithms: www.resus.org.uk

Resuscitation Council, *Advanced Life Support*, 6th edition, 2011, Resuscitation Council UK,

Chapter 28

British Medical Journal: www.bmj.com

Patient Safety: www.npsa.nhs.uk/alerts

Chapter 30

MedlinePlus: www.nlm.nih.gov

Chapter 32

Blundell A, Harrison R, *OSCE's at a Glance*, 2nd edition, 2013, Wiley Blackwell, Oxford.

Chapter 33

Gleadle J, *History and Examination at a Glance*, 3rd edition, 2012, Wiley Blackwell, Oxford.

Chapter 34

Donald A, Stein M, Scott Hill C, *The Hands-on Guide for Junior Doctors*, 4th edition, 2011, Wiley Blackwell, Oxford.

Dorries C, *Coroners' Court – a Guide to Law and Practice*, 2nd edition, 2004, Oxford University Press, Oxford.

Index

abbreviations, approved 25
absence of vital signs 91
acid–base status of blood 51
adhesive labels 11
adverse drug reactions 25
aerosol metered dose inhaler 54
airway adjuncts 58–9
airway manoeuvres 58–9
albumin 43
alcoholic gels 15
allergies 24
allergy 42
ampoules 45
anaemia 43
anaphylaxis 42
apnoea 61
aprons 15
arterial blood gas (ABG) measurement 50–51
arteriovenous fistula 29
asepsis 18–19
aseptic non-touch technique (ANTT) 18, 19
asthma 53
asystole 67
atrial depolarisation 65
atrial fibrillation 65
attentiveness 5
auscultation 23
automated external defibrillator (AED) 66
awareness of situations 4, 5

bag-valve mask ventilation 60–61
bag-valve masks 53, 61
barcodes for patient identification 11
bare below the elbow policy 15
basilic vein 28
bereavement officers 91
bereavement process 91
best interests of patients 13
best practice guidelines 11
bilirubin 77
black domestic waste disposal bins 7
bladder catheterisation 78–9
blood
    collection 29
    cultures 30–31
    donation 42, 43
    gas, arterial (ABG) 50–51
    gas, venous (VBG) 51
    glucose determination 34–5

intravenous infusions 42–3
    type compatibilities 42
    in urine 77
blood pressure 23
    determination 22
    hypertensive retinopathy 86
bloodborne infections 7
body language 5
Body Mass Index (BMI) 71
bolus doses 25
bradycardia 65
breaks from work 3
breath-actuated inhalers 54
British National Formulary (BNF) 25, 45

cannula insertion 32–3
capabilities, personal 3
capacity 13
cardiac monitoring 65
cardiopulmonary resuscitation (CPR) 66–7
care, personal 3
care, quality of 3, 4
catheter specimen of urine (CSU) 77
cephalic vein 28
certifying death 90–91
chaperones 5
Charrières catheter sizes 78–9
chin lift 58, 59
chronic obstructive pulmonary disorder (COPD) 25, 53, 54
ciliary muscle 87
cleanliness, importance of 7
clinical care 4, 17
clinical waste disposal 7
clothing, appropriate 5
colloids 41
communication 4, 5
companion website to this book xviii
competence in acting 3
complaints 13
confidence in acting 3
confidential waste disposal 7
confidentiality 5, 7
consent 12–13
contamination avoidance 7
Control of Substances Hazardous to Health (COSHH) 15
coroners 91
counselling for bereavement 91
Cremation Form 91
cross-matching blood 43
cryoprecipitate 43
crystalloids 41

Practical Medical Procedures at a Glance, First Edition. Rachel K. Thomas © Rachel K. Thomas. Published 2015 by John Wiley & Sons, Ltd.
Companion website: http://www.ataglanceseries.com/practicalmedprocedures

death certificates 90–91
decision making 4, 5
defibrillation 66, 67
dehydration 41
Department of Health best practice guidelines 11
deranged clotting 43
diabetes
    retinopathy 86, 87
    urine test strips 77
diabetic ketoacidosis (DKA) 34
diagnosis of conditions 3
diastolic blood pressure 23
dieticians 71
digital rectal examination (DRE) 72–3
diluents 25, 45
dipstick urine tests 76–7
disposable gloves 15
documentation 3
    importance of 13
domestic waste disposal 7
dorsal venous arch 28
dosage of drugs 24
drainage bag 70
dress, appropriate 5
drip arm 29
drug dosage 24
drug interactions 24
drug names 24
drug-related deaths 91
dry powdered inhalers (DPIs) 54

ear drum examination 82–3
ear grommets 82, 83
electrocardiogram (ECG) recordings 64–5
endotracheal tube 58
enteral nutrition bag 70
errors 5
exchange transfusions 43
experience 3
eye contact during communication 5
eyedrops 86

feedback and complaints 13
feeding 71
flame haemorrhages of the retina 87
fluid balance maintenance 25
fluid overload 42
forced expiratory capacity (FEC) 57
forced expiratory volume (FEV_1) 57
formal consent 12
fovea 87
Fraser competence 13
French gauge for catheter sizes 78–9
frequency of drug use 24
fresh frozen plasma 43
fundoscopy 87

General Medical Council (GMC) 3
    capacity 13
    Tomorrow's Doctors 3
Gillick competence 13
glaucoma 87

glucose measurement
    blood 34–5
    urine 77
gowns 15
guidance 3
guidelines, best practice 11

haematuria 77
haemolytic transfusion reaction 42
hair caps 15, 17
haloperidol injections 46
hand hygiene 14–15
head tilt 58, 59
healthcare-associated infections (HCAIs) 19
hearing loss 83
heart rate 23, 65
help, seeking 3
heparin injections 46
heparinised syringe 51
Her Majesty's (HM) Coroner 91
High Court decisions about intervention 12
high-flow oxygen 53
Hippocratic Oath 2, 3
human albumin 43
hypercapnic respiratory failure 53
hyperglycaemia 34, 35
hypertensive retinopathy 86
hypoglycaemia 34, 35
hypoventilation 61
hypoxemia 53

identifying the patient 5, 10–11
I-gel® airway 58
industry-related deaths 91
infection control 15, 17, 19
inhalers 25, 54–5
injections 46–7
insulin injections 46
Internet resources xviii
intervention, consent to 12
intradermal (ID) injections 46
intramuscular (IM) injections 46–7
intravenous (IV) fluids 25
intravenous (IV) infusions, administering 40–41
    blood/blood products 42–3
intravenous (IV) injections 47
introducing oneself 5, 11
invasive procedures
    patient identification 11
    scrubbing in 17

jaw thrust 58, 59

ketones 77

language use 5
laryngeal mask airway 58
leadership 4
leukocyte esterase 77
light reflex 83
limitations, personal 3
liver failure 24

local anaesthetic injections 46
location of consultations/questioning 5
long-term oxygen therapy (LTOT) 53

macula 87
malleus 83
management of conditions 3
masks 15, 17
median cubital vein 28
median vein 28
Medical Certificate of the Cause of Death (MCCD) 91
medical defence union 13
medication charts 3
Mental Capacity Act (2005) 13
metoclopramide injections 46
midstream urine (MSU) sample 77
modified early warning system (MEWS) 22, 23
multiple data points of identification 11

nasal cannulae 25, 53
nasogastric (NG) tubes 70–71
nasopharyngeal airways 58, 59
National Institute for Clinical Excellence (NICE) 25
nebulisers 25, 54–5
needle safe units 7
needle types 36, 37
neurological exam 87
never events, incorrect patient identification 11
nitrites 77
non-haemolytic transfusion reaction 42
non-rebreather masks 25, 53
non-shockable rhythms 67
non-technical skills 4–5
non-verbal communication 4, 5
notes, patient 5, 13, 25
nurses 3
nutrient deficiencies 71
nutritional assessment 71

oath of World Medical Association 2
observation charts 22
obstructive versus restrictive respiratory disorders 56
Occupational Health for sharps injuries 7
open-ended questions 5, 11
ophthalmoscopy 86–7
optic atrophy 87
optimum outcomes 5
oral glucose tolerance test 35
order of draw for blood sample 29
oropharyngeal airways 58
otalgia 83
otitis media 82, 83
otorrhoea 83
otoscopy 82–3
overfilling of waste bins 7
oxygen
    high-flow 53
    prescribing 25
oxygen saturation 23
oxygen saturation probe 22
oxygen therapy, administering 52–3
oxygen therapy concentration (FiO$_2$) 51

P wave 64
packed red cells 43
PaCO$_2$ 51
pamphlets 5
PaO$_2$ 51
papilloedema 86
parental responsibility 13
parenteral medications, administering 44–5
patient capacity 13
patient care, quality of 3
patient-controlled analgesia (PCA) 25
patient identification 10–11
patient moving equipment 3
patient notes 5, 13, 25
patient rights 13
patient safety rights 10, 11
patient support groups 5
patients with similar/same names, avoiding confusion 11
peak expiratory flow respiration 57
peak flow respiration 57
per rectum (PR) 73
percutaneous endoscopic gastrostomy (PEG) 71
perforated tympanic membrane 82
permission from patients 12
personal protective equipment (PPE) 14–15
pH
    blood 51
    urine 77
planning 5
plasma glucose measurement 34–5
platelets 43
plethysmography 57
portable sharps bins 7
PR interval 64
practical procedures 2–3
preparation 5
prescriptions 24–5
privacy of patients 5
Procurator Fiscal (Scotland) 91
prostate gland palpation 72, 73
proteins in urine 77
proteinuria 77
protocols 3
pulseless electrical activity (PEA) 67
pumps for IV infusions 41

QRS complex 64
QT interval 64
quality patient care 3
quick response (QR) codes for patient identification 11

rectal examination, digital (DRE) 72–3
recycling waste 7
red reflex 87
referrals 5
Registrar of Births and Deaths 91
regular medications 25
renal failure 24
respiratory function assessment 56–7
respiratory rate 23
resting 3
restrictive versus obstructive respiratory disorders 56

retina 86, 87
risk assessment for sharps injuries 7
route of administration 24
RR interval 64
Ryle's tube 70

safe practice 3
safety rights of patients 10, 11
scrubbing in/up 16–17
sepsis 30, 31
septic screen 23
sharps injuries 7
sharps waste, safe disposal of 7
single-use gloves 15
sinus rhythm 65
site practitioners 3
situation awareness 4, 5
six steps of hand washing 14, 15
sketches 5
sphygmomanometer use 23
spirometry 57
ST segment 64
staples 37
stat dosage 25
steri-strips 37
stethoscope use 23
stress 4
subcutaneous (SC) injections 46, 47
suicides, reporting 91
support groups for patients 5
surgical scrubbing 17
suspicious cause of death 91
suturing 36–7
    suture types 37
swabs 19
syringe drivers 25
systolic blood pressure 23

T wave 64
tachycardia 65
task management 4, 5
teamwork 4
temperature measurement 22–3
test strips 76–7
theatre procedures 17
three-point identification of patients 11
three-way catheters 78
tidal volume flow 57
tinnitus 83
Tomorrow's Doctors (GMC) 3
total lung capacity 57

total parenteral nutrition (TPN) 71
tourniquet 29, 31
translators 5
treatment refusal, capacity for 13
tropicamide 87
two-point identification of patients 11
two-way Foley catheters 78
tympanic membrane 82
tympanic thermometers 22, 23

U wave 64
umbo 83
unconscious patients, identification
    of 11
universal donor blood 43
unknown cause of death 91
unnatural death 91
urinalysis 76–7
urinary tract infections (UTIs) 77
urine, colour of 77
urobilinogen 77

Vacutainer® needle 29, 31
venepuncture 28–9
venous blood gas (VBG) 51
ventricular fibrillation (VF) 67
ventricular tachycardia (VT) 67
Venturi adaptors and flow rates 52
Venturi mask 25, 53
verbal communication 4, 5
verbal consent 12
vertigo 83
vials 45
Visual Infusion Phlebitis (VIP) score 32
vital capacity 57
vital sign measurement 22–3
vital signs, absence of 91

waste disposal 6–7
website accompanying this book xviii
workspace modification 5
World Medical Association oath 2
wristbands for patient identification 11
written communication 4, 5
written consent 12

xiphisternum 70

Yellow Card scheme 25
yellow clinical sharps bins 7
yellow clinical waste bins 7

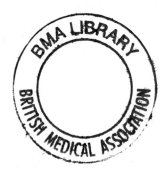